NURSING LEADERSHIP AND MANAGEMENT SKILLS

TO ACCOMPANY

LEADING AND MANAGING IN NURSING
YODER WISE

Mary J. Keenan, R.N., Ph.D.
Associate Professor
Medical College of Ohio
School of Nursing
Toledo, Ohio

Joseph B. Hurst, Ph.D., Ed.D.
Professor
University of Toledo
College of Education and Allied Professions
Toledo, Ohio

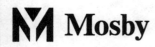 Mosby

St. Louis Baltimore Boston Carlsbad Chicago Naples New York Philadelphia Portland
London Madrid Mexico City Singapore Sydney Tokyo Toronto Wiesbaden

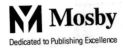

Mosby

Dedicated to Publishing Excellence

Publisher: Nancy L. Coon
Executive Editor: Darlene Como
Developmental Editor: Dana Knighten
Project Manager: Chris Baumle
Production Editor: Stacy M. Guarracino
Designer: Nancy McDonald
Manufacturing Supervisor: Karen Lewis

FIRST EDITION
COPYRIGHT © 1995 BY MOSBY–YEAR BOOK, INC.
A Mosby imprint of Mosby–Year Book, Inc.

Printed in the United States of America

Mosby–Year Book, Inc.
11830 Westline Industrial Drive
St. Louis, Missouri 63146

International Standard Book Number 0-8151-5207-8

This workbook has been developed to promote learning, recall, and clinical application of leadership and management principles discussed in *Leading and Managing in Nursing*. Faculty who teach management have collaborated with their peers and colleagues in nursing service, business, and continuing education to produce this workbook. Through our collective knowledge and experience, we have developed varied exercises to use (independently and in groups) to illustrate the concepts and theories of management.

Since we all learn in different ways, at different paces, and in different modes, the exercises in this workbook have been designed to meet individual and group learning needs. We have selected recurring themes and case studies that we believe are significant in management practice and have incorporated them throughout the workbook.

We believe that as clinical practice changes, so does the application of management concepts and theories. An excellent clinician is not necessarily an excellent manager, and the reverse is also true. This book focuses on clinical management; therefore, the applications call forth self-awareness, abilities, and skills in working with patients, families, nurses, and colleagues in other disciplines to achieve patient care goals. We acknowledge the rapidly evolving changes in healthcare delivery and have included exercises in managing dilemmas, communicating, and using group skills.

Recognizing that not all learning takes place in the classroom, we have included exercises that can be used either in class or outside of class. We have also developed some exercises that can be used to plan for clinical experiences and some that can help in developing individualized clinical management objectives. Since we believe strongly that the input of practicing professionals is critical to providing students with a realistic learning experience, we have included exercises that request feedback from nursing staff members and one exercise that is devoted to offering positively framed feedback to our invaluable mentors in nursing services. We hope you have as much fun working through these exercises as we did in developing them.

We would like to acknowledge the contributions of Bonnie Nelson, M.S.N., R.N., not only as a contributor to this workbook, but also for her invaluable contributions in the final preparation of this manuscript. Her careful, caring commentary throughout and her direct assistance in assembling the final manuscript have expedited the completion of this workbook.

Mary J. Keenan, R.N., Ph.D.
Joseph B. Hurst, Ph.D., Ed.D.

CONTRIBUTORS

Paula Bonell, B.S.N., R.N.
Graduate Student, Medical College of Ohio

Ann W. Baker, Ph.D., R.N.
Assistant Professor, Medical College of Ohio

Marsha Brown, M.S.N., R.N.
Visiting Nurse Service, Toledo, Ohio

Marcy R. Bugajski, B.S.N., R.N.
Graduate Student, Medical College of Ohio

Mary Ann Dimmick, M.S.N., R.N.
Nursing Director, Medical College Hospitals

Mary Beth Hayward, M.S.N., R.N.
Assistant Professor, Medical College of Ohio

Rosemary Kahle, M.Ed., R.N.
Assistant Professor, Medical College of Ohio

Tim Krzys, M.S.N., R.N.
Rehabilitation Specialist

Bonnie Nelson, M.S.N., R.N.
Instructor, Medical College of Ohio

Rosalind M. Peters, M.S.N., R.N.
Assistant Professor, Medical College of Ohio

Neil VanderVeen, Ph.D.
Assistant Professor, University of Toledo

TABLE OF CONTENTS

PART 1
MANAGING AND LEADING:
THE CONCEPTS

CHAPTER 1

MANAGING AND LEADING

Mary J. Keenan, Ph.D., R.N., Joseph B. Hurst,
Ph.D., Ed.D., and Tim Krzys, M.S.N., R.N.

INTRODUCTION

It has been said that an effective *manager* focuses efficiently on objectives, tasks, procedures, and policies. But recently, the emphasis has been on *leaders* who provide vision, inspiration, and empowerment. Exactly what does each of these terms mean? Who should lead, manage, or follow, and when? The activities in this chapter are designed to help you recognize the differences between leading and managing and to recognize how and why both behaviors are essential for organizations to move forward.

OBJECTIVES

- To identify differences in the roles, activities, specific behaviors, and outcomes of managing and leading.

- To identify how each contributes to the mission and goals of a healthcare institution.

- To determine what might happen if there is management without leadership and leadership without management in an organization or group.

- To apply the techniques of mindmapping to studying, to make relevant meaning of leadership theory, and to apply new skills to real-life situations.

1. Make a list of essential managing and leading tasks (e.g., page 7 in the text) that are important to your own development by completing the two lists of verbs below.

MANAGING TASKS

a) Plan

b) Organize

c)

d)

e)

f)

LEADING TASKS

a) Envision

b) Inspire

c)

d)

e)

f)

2. In the space below or on another piece of paper make another list of leading and managing tasks in which you are already engaged in some aspects of your life.

PRESENT LEADING TASKS   **PRESENT MANAGING TASKS**

3. Now that you have derived a list of managing and leading tasks relevant to you, list one specific behavior you could develop and use for each of the tasks that you have cited above.

MANAGING BEHAVIORS

a) Do an outline of the project by tomorrow

b)

c)

d)

e)

f)

LEADING BEHAVIORS

a) Envision/dream how to do things differently

b)

c)

d)

e)

f)

ACTIVITY 1–2

Write a short analysis of the similarities and differences among managers and leaders on a unit of a hospital with which you are familiar. Discuss these similarities and differences with others (staff nurses, nurse managers, and other students).

ACTIVITY 1–3

1. In the spaces below, write a list of the positive consequences (beneficial outcomes) that occur when one manages well and when one leads well.

Beneficial Outcomes or Consequences

MANAGING WELL	LEADING WELL
a) Orderly, organized unit	a) Progressive, creative unit
b)	b)
c)	c)
d)	d)
e)	e)
f)	f)

2. Write any observations, questions, and/or conclusions you have about the above two lists.

3. Write a list of the negative consequences/outcomes of (or difficulties caused by) overemphasizing managing to the exclusion of leading, and then overemphasizing leading to the exclusion of managing.

Negative Outcomes or Consequences

OVEREMPHASIZING MANAGING	OVEREMPHASIZING LEADING
a) Limited freedom for staff	a) Out of touch with reality
b)	b)
c)	c)
d)	d)
e)	e)

4. Write any questions, observations, and/or conclusions you have about the above two lists.

5. Discuss with at least one other person the benefits and negative results (all four lists) of leading and managing. List specific ways you could (or have seen others) shift emphasis between leading and managing.
   a) What behaviors, policies, procedures, etc. facilitate a shift of emphasis from managing to leading and back again IN THE INSTITUTION(S) YOU HAVE CHOSEN?

   b) What behaviors, policies, procedures, etc. block this shifting emphasis IN THE INSTITUTION(S) YOU HAVE CHOSEN?

   c) What new behaviors, policies, procedures, etc. would produce an effective shifting in the future IN THE INSTITUTION(S) YOU HAVE CHOSEN?

ACTIVITY 1–4

Read at least three articles concerning managing and leading. Notice the degree to which the articles focus on the benefits of either leading or managing and the consequences of the other. When this occurs the article tends to be a "crusade" for one side of this dilemma as though the author's favored approach is the solution to a particular problem. By overemphasizing the favored side, you could eventually experience its negative consequences, just as walking along one side of a seesaw will at some point make it tip downward (see your negative consequences listed above). Do any of your articles call for both leading and managing together, or mix them into a "superperson" profile? This may lead to clouding the distinctions and ignoring the need to emphasize leading or managing when appropriate.

1. What do the articles recommend about shifting focus?

2. With what level of certainty do the authors speak about the most needed behaviors?

3. What recommendations could you use in your clinical or work setting?

4. Why?

1. Team up with another student in your class. Separately, compile a list of what you each believe are leadership behaviors. Try to list at least ten.

2. Review your lists, and mark your initials beside each behavior that you believe can be used to describe some of your own behaviors. Do this without input from anyone else. Using the same lists, indicate by marking your partner's initials which behaviors you have observed in the other student. Do this activity without any input from the other student. When finished, compare lists.

3. What do you both notice about the differences in how you view yourselves and how you view one another?

4. What did you learn about yourselves?

5. Do others see you as having more, or fewer, leadership traits than you believe you have? Why?

MINDMAPPING: A CREATIVE APPROACH TO THINKING

According to Wycoff (1991) mindmapping is a technique that fosters creative thinking through logical and convergent abilities on the one hand and imaginative and divergent abilities on the other. Mindmapping could be viewed as an open, visually driven way to outline a number of different tasks including solving problems, organizing and completing projects, listing tasks, accomplishing results, writing reports that need organization and depth, brainstorming new possibilities, making meetings and note taking more effective, developing and delivering important presentations, and promoting personal growth and planning (Wycoff, pp.41–42). The sample mindmap in Figure 1-1 below illustrates the basic elements of this process.

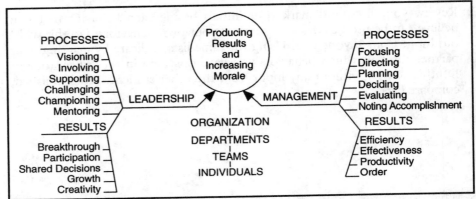

Figure 1-1   Sample mindmap.

THE MINDMAPPING PROCESS

There are some very basic, simple steps to take to develop your own mindmap for almost any purpose. First, decide on the central focus of the map and draw or stick a colorful image, symbol, or graphic in the center of a large sheet of paper, white or black board, poster board, or chart pad sheet. This is a vital step in the process. Wycoff suggests that people consider the main focus carefully, and jot down different possibilities until an appropriate focus is determined, one that is expansive enough to foster creativity and yet relevant to the desired results.

Second, focus your attention on this central "figure/topic" and allow your thinking to flow without restrictions, judgments, and order. This involves practice in letting go of limiting thoughts and habits so you can explore your mind and thinking fully.

Third, represent ideas by jotting down one or two words someplace on the map. Wycoff recommends one key word/phrase per line, using color and visuals to highlight key ideas on your maps.

Fourth, connect the key words to the central focus with lines. Continue to look for patterns, especially new ones.

Mindmapping has several uses. Throughout this book you will find exercises that ask you to create, revise, and use mindmaps of chapter content, leadership and management skills, personal and institutional visions and goals, professional and personal problems and projects, plans and meetings, conflicts and dilemmas, and legal and ethical issues.

ACTIVITY 1–7

Taking Chapter 1 entirely as your focus, or some important ideas/skills from the chapter, create a mindmap of your own sense of the chapter's meaning and applications to real life.

REFERENCE

Wycoff, J. (1991). Mindmapping: Your personal guide to exploring creativity and problem–solving. New York: Berkley Books.

CHAPTER 2

THE ROLE OF NURSE MANAGER

Marsha Brown, M.S.N., R.N., and Mary Ann Dimmick, M.S.N., R.N.

INTRODUCTION

So you want to be a nurse manager? If so, you are studying a very challenging aspect of the nursing profession. Actually, it's much like having entered a juggling contest. You will learn to "juggle" budgets and staff for patient needs, to be a resource person for clinical expertise, and to act as a change agent. These roles may seem confusing, challenging, or conflicting at times, but there are many rewards.

The following experiences have been developed for you by people who have been or now are nurse managers. We hope that they are of benefit to you as you learn about the many role relationships required in the position.

OBJECTIVES

* To identify and examine many of the diverse roles and responsibilities of a nurse manager.

* To practice some of these roles and responsibilities and give/receive feedback about the actions taken.

ACTIVITY 2-1

SCENARIO A: THE UNHAPPY CAMPER

You've just been handed a stack of staff nurse performance evaluations by your superior. You must have them done in one month. You very carefully spend a seemingly inordinate amount of time on each evaluation, taking great pains to be as objective and diplomatic as you can possibly be. Like some good managers, you do the easier ones first, saving the difficult ones for last. You complete all but the last evaluation. This particular staff nurse is not a "happy camper," to say the least. You want to focus on strengths as well as areas for improvement so you can develop a plan for improvement with this staff nurse. Good luck!

1. To prepare for writing the evaluation, you have determined that you need to identify specific instances (critical incidents) that led you to the conclusion of "unhappy camper." Cite some specific examples or instances that would support this conclusion. Here are a few; add others from your experiences with unhappy campers with whom you have worked:

   a) Frequent grumbling about things that do not go as expected, with no apparent commitment to do anything about it.

   b) Seldom offers assistance to other staff.

   c)

   d)

   e)

2. Cite some positive examples or instances that do not support this conclusion and reflect positive behaviors and outcomes.

   a) Well liked by patients as seen in their comments on written surveys or evaluations.

   b) Always punctual.

   c)

   d)

   e)

3. Develop two critical incident reports based on each of the two above scenarios that you have generated, i.e., the "unhappy camper" and the positive supportive behavioral example. A critical incident report is a detailed written description of one event in which the employee was involved. The key word is *descriptive*. Focus on what happened, what was said, and how the employee behaved. You may wish to include more than one behavior in the critical incident. Do not attempt to include all of them. Make up these incidents or use ones you recall.

CRITICAL INCIDENT: UNHAPPY CAMPER

CRITICAL INCIDENT: POSITIVE SUPPORTIVE BEHAVIORS

What do you notice about your writing of these incidents? What could you do to improve your abilities to do this?

ACTIVITY 2-2

In Chapter 2 in the textbook, interdependency and delegation are discussed as important aspects of the nurse manager's role. This activity focuses on the blocks to and necessary elements of effective delegating.

Read the list of common blocks to delegating and check (✓) those that pertain to your own ability to delegate to others.

BLOCKS TO EFFECTIVE DELEGATING

___ 1. I can do it better myself.

___ 2. I lack confidence in others' abilities.

___ 3. I tend to be a perfectionist.

___ 4. I'm not secure in my role.

___ 5. I prefer to manage every detail of projects.

___ 6. I have not trained others to do it.

___ 7. I have a habit of overworking (doing it all myself).

___ 8. I tend to assist others with their work.

___ 9. My backlog of work doesn't give me enough time to delegate effectively.

___ 10. I still prefer to do most of the work.

___ 11. I'm usually rushing to meet my schedule and deadlines.

___ 12. I do not trust others' competency enough.

___ 13. Explaining work to others is too difficult.

___ 14. Others are so busy that I'm afraid they won't like me or would be angry if I gave them more work.

___ 15. I just can't let go of even less-important responsibilities.

___ 16. It's just much easier to do it myself.

___ 17. If others did it better than I do, then I could lose my job or look less competent.

___ 18. Although others are able, I don't believe they will be responsible enough to do it on time.

SUMMARY: Looking at your pattern of check marks above, what observations and conclusions can you make?

Read the list of elements of effective delegating below and check those you already do when you delegate and star (*) those you could start to use as you increase and improve your delegating.

ELEMENTS OF EFFECTIVE DELEGATING

___ 1. Identify the "big picture" or overall rationale and priorities.

___ 2. Specify the task clearly.

___ 3. Designate a sufficient time deadline.

___ 4. Communicate fully and often.

___ 5. Delegate to someone who can and will do the job.

___ 6. Request, attend to, and act on progress reports.

___ 7. Provide and clarify any direction needed.

___ 8. First, delegate things you do well, if appropriate.

___ 9. Then, delegate tasks/projects that take you a great deal of time and energy.

___ 10. Encourage others and acknowledge progress and effort without "checking up."

___ 11. Provide and/or make available resources necessary to complete the task/project well.

___ 12. Clarify the scope of others' responsibility and accountability while stressing excellence.

___ 13. Explain the purposes and priority of the tasks.

___ 14. Remember to delegate the results to be produced for which you and others are being held accountable.

___ 15. Assist others in setting targeted, realistic deadlines and follow up checkpoints in time.

SUMMARY: Look over your pattern of responses above. What important observations, conclusions, and new commitments can you make about your own delegating?

Read the scenario below and consider what you have read in Chapters 1 and 2 in your textbook. Answer the questions specifically as if you were the nurse manager in this case.

SCENARIO B: WHAT DOES THIS REALLY COST?

The newly appointed medical director of the unit that you manage (whom you have just met) has requested a new, expensive piece of equipment. You know your budget has already been established for the fiscal year and you also know that this request is not cost-effective. In fact, if adopted this request also will be more labor intensive for the nursing staff.

1. How could you say "no" without creating defensiveness?

2. How could you say "no" while leaving the "maybe there are other possibilities" option open?

ACTIVITY 2-4

Observational experience: As a part of your clinical experiences, you usually have the opportunity to be with a nurse manager in some capacity.

Objective: To identify at least three specific interactions between the manager and others (staff, physicians, yourself, etc.). For example, consider a manager and a nurse in the nourishment room at 9:20 A.M. Subject: a scheduling conflict. Activities:

1. Briefly summarize each interaction in one paragraph in your notebook or diary.

2. Cite the leadership style(s) used by the manager in each situation.

3. Identify other nurse manager roles and responsibilities in these three situations cited above. What would be some of the behaviors you would have to demonstrate in those situations?

4. Compare and contrast these examples with specific selected readings from your textbook Chapters 1 and 2.

ACTIVITY 2-5

MINDMAPPING

1. Create a mindmap of Chapter 2 in your textbook.
2. In the previous chapter you were asked to complete a mindmapping exercise. If you completed that map, look at it now and see how you would integrate the additional ideas and skills from Chapter 2. Also add more symbols and visuals to your mapping, and ask others outside the class to do some mindmapping with you and give you their input.

CHAPTER 3

LEGAL AND ETHICAL ISSUES

Bonnie Nelson, M.S.N., R.N.

INTRODUCTION

The increasing demands in healthcare for cost containment and quality in patient care services, combined with increasing technology, pose escalating ethical and legal questions. As the healthcare scene changes, so do the questions that are posed to staff nurses and managers. This chapter presents dilemmas that can assist in heightening your awareness of legal and ethical issues that are prominent today. This chapter provides not answers but rather ideas for further inquiry. These exercises are designed to offer you an opportunity to try out and to experience some of the dilemmas that are posed to managers and staff. The exercises were selected as representative of current examples of common dilemmas that you may encounter.

OBJECTIVES

- **To determine factors to be considered in assignment of personnel who have been cross-trained.**

- **To distinguish between the information reported on a patient's chart and that on the incident report following an occurrence.**

- **To determine your position on a required request from the perspective of deontological and/or teleological theories.**

- **To evaluate an ethical dilemma using the MORAL model.**

ACTIVITY 3–1

You are the charge nurse on a medical surgical unit and have been requested to send an RN to the coronary care unit because one of the nurses there must leave. The charge nurse on the coronary care unit calls you a few minutes later after the RN arrives from the medical surgical unit and is requesting that you and she talk with the nurse who has changed units. You go to the conference room and the RN immediately complains that it was her turn to be pulled but that she has never been trained in critical care and is afraid that she will lose her license if she does something wrong while working there. Furthermore, there was another RN who has had intensive care unit experience, but she would not go because it was "not her turn to be pulled."

1. How would you respond to the RN who has been pulled?

2. Would you request the other RN, even though it was not her turn? Provide a rationale.

3. Could cross–training have eliminated this dilemma?

4. Consider what units in your institution might logically be identified for cross–training? State the rationale.
   a) Units:
   b) Rationale:

5. What would be involved in cross–training, and what levels of personnel would be involved?
   a) What is involved:

   b) Personnel level(s):

6. Take a position—cross–training does or does not reduce costs?

ACTIVITY 3–2

An alternate definition of cross–training is the training of personnel with different educational backgrounds to perform tasks often performed by another. Using this definition, consider the situation in Activity 3–1 and resolve the staffing problem. Provide a rationale for your resolutions. Include any new dilemmas that are created by the use of this definition of cross–training.

1. Could the clerical specialist be trained to do vital signs or collect and calculate intake and output?

2. Could the nursing assistant collect blood specimens?

3. Could the respiratory therapist be responsible for turning and positioning the patient that he is suctioning every two hours?

4. Do any of these resolutions violate the nurse practice act in your state? Discuss.

As nurse manager it is your responsibility to review all incidents that occur on your unit to determine if they were reported according to protocol and if appropriate follow–up has been completed.

On the previous day, one patient received injuries to her hand while ambulating when an IV controller slipped on the IV pole and pinned her hand between the controller and a platform designed to be used as a flat surface to hold equipment while working with the IV.

The incident report states: "Patient was ambulating to bathroom at 10:30 P.M. and used the IV pole to stabilize herself while walking. The controller fell down the pole and pinned her right hand to the small table beneath it. Injury evident to right hand. Hand immediately began to swell and patient had acute pain. X–ray revealed a fracture of the third and fourth metacarpal of the right hand. Physician notified, responded, and orthopedic consult ordered."

The nurse's note in the chart states: "Patient ambulating to bathroom using IV pole to stabilize herself. IV controller fell, pinning hand, resulting in injury. This would not have happened if I had been present to help her. She stated that she turned on her light but no one answered because the unit was very busy at the time. Physician notified and responded. Incident report filed."

1. Identify and examine potential liability from this incident.

2. How does the note made in the chart affect the potential liability for a) the nurse involved, b) the nurse manager, and c) the institution.
   a) nurse

   b) nurse manager

   c) institution

3. Rewrite the nurse's note.

ACTIVITY 3–4

Required Request has been made into law in many states. This law requires that after all deaths the family must be made aware of the possibility of donation of organs and tissues.

1. Identify the values and beliefs of Required Request from both the deontological and the teleological perspectives.

    a) Deontological

    b) Teleological

2. Identify your position regarding Required Request. Do you more closely follow the deontological or the teleological perspective? State three reasons to support your position.

    Position

    a)

    b)

    c)

You are the nurse manager on a busy intermediate coronary care unit. You have just received a request from the admitting department for a bed on your unit, but there are no beds available. You inform the admitting department and request more information on the patient. The information you receive is that the patient is a 73-year-old woman with congestive heart failure who needs to receive IV medications. The doctor has requested that she be on a monitored bed while receiving the medication. After reviewing all of the patients on the unit, it is decided to transfer a 48-year-old man who had a myocardial infarction six days earlier and who is being discharged tomorrow. The patient is transferred and you receive the woman with congestive heart failure. The next day you find out that during the night the patient who was transferred was found in complete arrest when the nurse on the other unit made rounds at 2:00 A.M. The man was resuscitated but is now in intensive care with brain damage resulting from the anoxia that occurred before he was resuscitated.

1. Was the decision to transfer the patient out of the intermediate care unit appropriate? Provide a rationale for your answer.

2. Use the MORAL model discussed in the textbook to review this ethical dilemma.
   M   Massage the dilemma; identify and define the issues in the dilemma.

O   Outline the options.

R   Resolve the dilemma.

A   Act by applying the chosen option.

L   Look back and evaluate the entire process.

You are caring for Mrs. Jacobs and she has asked to review her medical record. It is within the law of your state for patients to have the right of access to the chart while they are hospitalized. You are supervising Mrs. Jacobs during the review of her record.

Mrs. Jacobs is very upset when she sees that one of the nurses on the previous night documented that she was crying and seemed depressed after her family left. She states she doesn't have any problems with her family and does not want anyone to think she is depressed because she doesn't want to see a psychiatrist. She is demanding that the charting be changed because she wasn't depressed.

1. Can you legally alter the charting that another nurse has done? Provide a rationale.

2. How can you explain this to Mrs. Jacobs?

3. How would you respond to Mrs. Jacobs when she says that if you do not change the note that she is calling her attorney?

4. Write an example of a nurse's note to reflect the observations of the nurse without the inference of depression.

ACTIVITY 3–7

MINDMAPPING

Create a mindmap of Chapter 3 in the textbook, using visuals and symbols where you think they are appropriate. Try to integrate the "Terms to Know" from the text's "Chapter Checklist" into your mindmap so that you can use it as a test review aid.

CHAPTER 4

STRATEGIC PLANNING, GOAL SETTING, AND MARKETING

Neil VanderVeen, Ph.D.

INTRODUCTION

In Chapter 4 in the textbook, you have been learning the importance of planning strategically, developing clear goals and objectives, implementing in a disciplined manner, and marketing concepts in the field of healthcare. You have also considered the critical importance of integrating the planning, targeting, implementing, and marketing functions. This chapter provides processes to enable you to develop skills in performing these functions.

OBJECTIVES

- To be able to use and assess an established tool for assessing the level of planning, targeting, implementing, and marketing in an organization.

- To provide a structure for practicing the strategic planning process in a group context.

- To increase, through practice, the ability to write clear goals and objectives based on a strategic plan.

- To develop the ability to clearly assess marketing challenges.

ACTIVITY 4-1

1. To identify the marketing strategies of a healthcare organization obtain a copy of at least one marketing brochure or plan for your own organization or one with which you are familiar.

2. Analyze the completeness and effectiveness of your brochure or plan according to the following criteria:

   a) Is the market for each product or service clearly defined?

   b) Are organization resources (capacity to deliver the product or service) quantified for each product or service?

   c) What are the marketing objectives? Are they realistic, specific, measurable, and mutually consistent?

   d) Are specific market segments identified for increased penetration?

   e) Is the planned mix of products and services clearly defined or will the mix be reactive to market requirements?

Select a healthcare organization and assess its current state with regard to the planning, targeting, implementing, and marketing functions. You can conduct this type of assessment by reviewing such relevant documents in the organization as mission statements, strategic plans, tentative budgets, etc. In reviewing documents, what would you use as review criteria? List those criteria below.

REVIEWING THE STRATEGIC PLAN

Review Criteria	Not Met	Partly Met	Fully Met
1.			
2.			
3.			

Checking Your Thinking: Do your review criteria include the steps listed in the textbook? What are the practical implications of your answer?

REVIEWING GOALS AND OBJECTIVES

Review Criteria	Not Met	Partly Met	Fully Met
1.			
2.			
3.			

Checking Your Thinking: Do your review criteria include the steps listed in the textbook? What are the practical implications of your answer?

REVIEWING THE MARKETING PLAN

Review Criteria	Not Met	Partly Met	Fully Met
1.			
2.			
3.			

Checking Your Thinking: Does your review criteria include the steps listed in the textbook? What are the practical implications of your answer?

ACTIVITY 4-3

1. Participate in independent activity or small group discussion with students outside of class

2. The case study in the textbook (Chapter 4 Appendix) lists four forthcoming changes and develops a strategic planning document that responds to those changes. With your group members, discuss (or reflect by yourself on) how the plan would have to be altered if the changes included the following, rather than those mentioned in the case:

   a) Shared governance

   b) Program management (or case management)

   c) Reduction in budgets

   d) Increased regulation by government and professional associations

3. What are the main principles inherent in the concepts of budget reductions and increased regulation?

   Checking Your Thinking: Are the principles you have developed comprehensive? Are the statements concise and easily understood?

ACTIVITY 4-4

Planning is a critically important function. Without plans, we cannot sustain long-term initiatives. But planning must exist within a context of spontaneity, just as spontaneity must exist within a context of planning. To value one and eliminate the other will lead to system dysfunction!

1. List the benefits of planning.

2. List the problems associated with planning. Think about the problems that would occur if everything were planned and people were prohibited from taking any spontaneous action.

3. List the benefits associated with spontaneous action.

4. List the problems associated with spontaneous action. Think about the problems that would occur if no one in the organization did any planning.

Checking Your Thinking: See if your responses are similar to these benefits of planning:
- Enables allocation of resources
- Enables people to follow a common direction
- Provides a basis for performance measurement
- Enables long-term, proactive focus

Some problems of planning that is overdone and excludes spontaneity:
- Leads to organizational rigidity
- Impedes quick response to market changes
- Hinders individual creativity

Typical benefits of spontaneity:
- Allows for short-term flexibility
- Allows quick response to market changes
- Facilitates increased individual creativity

Some problems of spontaneity that is overdone and excludes planning:
- Impedes rational resource allocation
- Has no common direction
- Has no basis for performance measurement
- Has no basis for long-term focus

ACTIVITY 4-5

Planning requires effective vision, goals, and objectives. The textbook discusses guidelines for effective goals on page 71. Using these guidelines and examples write some specific short-term, medium range, and long-term goals for a department or team. Discuss them with another student and revise them as needed.

ACTIVITY 4-6

MINDMAPPING

1. Create a mindmap of Chapter 4 in your textbook.
2. Planning is an excellent activity in which to use mindmapping. Wycoff (1991, p. 91) suggests that people mindmap their goals using different colored pens for short-term, medium range, and long-term goals. Do this for Activity 4-5 or create a new map for your personal goals. Note any conflicts and barriers to these goals and add action plans (steps toward goal accomplishment) to this map.

CHAPTER 5

LEADING CHANGE: CONTINUITY OR CONFUSION

Neil VanderVeen, Ph.D.

INTRODUCTION

You have been studying the change process in terms of its stages, resistance to change, principles of effective change advocacy, and strategies to plan and manage change. This chapter provides structured opportunities to explore some of the dynamics of change.

OBJECTIVES

- To increase the ability to anticipate, and thus to plan for, resistance to change.

- To develop an understanding of change within the context of stability.

- To increase the ability to analyze a particular change process so that weaknesses can be identified.

ACTIVITY 5-1

Many organizations undergo so much change that people in the organizations cannot keep track of all that is changing. It is important to notice change so that we don't become desensitized to it. If we become desensitized, we take change for granted and fail to plan carefully for change initiatives. Identify the changes that have taken place in the healthcare organizations where you have worked or have had a clinical experience during the last one or two years. Think of what the organization, department, or work unit was trying to move away from and trying to move toward. An example might be moving away from centralized control and moving toward departmental control, or completing various quality improvement projects. Have some people at work assist you to build your list. Perhaps you could interview a staff nurse and/or manager. Write down as specifically as possible for each situation what people were moving away from and what they were moving toward.

MOVING AWAY FROM   **MOVING TOWARD**

ACTIVITY 5-2

Select one of the changes from the list below and analyze the change in terms of how it was presented to the potential adopters.

- Was a credible change agent used?

- Was it introduced on a trial basis?

- Was the relative advantage (to the adopters) clearly explained?

- Was there an attempt to make the benefits visible?

- Was the change compatible with beliefs and values of the adopters?

- Was there an attempt to reduce the apparent complexity?

- Was the change introduced during relative stability?

- With the benefit of hindsight, which of the above is most amenable to improvement?

- What actions would you recommend to make the improvement?

ACTIVITY 5-3

Many people believe that "it's just human nature to resist change." But this is an oversimplification of a complex issue. We can all think of changes that we would resist. We can also think of many changes that we would heartily endorse. Whether we resist or endorse a particular change depends on a number of variables. List below as many variables as you can think of that may affect whether you would resist or endorse a particular change.

Checking Your Thinking

1. The textbook refers to innovators, early adopters, and so on. Where a person falls on this scale is one variable.

2. The textbook also refers to characteristics of the change agent. These characteristics can have a powerful affect on whether people accept or reject change.

3. Everett Rogers (1983) discusses five characteristics of the innovation itself that will affect its rate of adoption.
   a) Relative advantage: "What's in it for me?"
   b) Trialability: "Can I adopt it on a trial basis?"
   c) Observability: "Can I see the benefits clearly and quickly?"
   d) Complexity: "How complicated will it be to adopt?"
   e) Compatibility: "Does the change fit with my values and beliefs?"

4. A particular change may be resistant because the level of change in general is too great. For example, I may reject a job offer from a different employer if my spouse and I are:
   a) expecting our first child,
   b) learning how to cope with caring for an aging parent, and
   c) preparing to move into a new house, all at the same time.

ACTIVITY 5-4

A particular change may be resisted because the level of change in general is too great. For example, I may reject a job offer from a different employer if my spouse and I are expecting our first child, learning how to cope with caring for an aging parent, and preparing to move into a new house, all at the same time. Item 4 under "Checking Your Thinking" on page 42 suggests a need to look at change in light of stability and to look at stability in the light of change. This is not an "either/or" issue! We cannot say that change is good or stability is bad. Nor can we say that stability is good or change is bad. They must be seen in relation to each other.

1. List the benefits of change. Don't focus on a specific change but think about change in general.

2. List some problems associated with change. Think about the problems that would occur if we always changed everything, if nothing were stable.

3. List some generic benefits of stability.

4. List the problems associated with stability. Think about the problems we would have if we never changed anything.

Checking Your Thinking: See if your responses are similar to the following:

Benefits of change:

- Ability to capitalize on new opportunities

- Excitement of new challenges

- Freedom from having to repeat mistakes

- Personal and organizational growth

Problems if change is overdone:

- Inability to train in a process before it changes

- Inability to perfect a process

- Exhaustion from too many new challenges

- Inability to develop and implement a plan

Benefits of stability:

- Staying with a process long enough to perfect it

- Ability to train people in processes

- Time to rest between new challenges

- Ability to develop a plan and to see it through

Problems if stability is overdone:

- Cannot capitalize on new opportunities

- No new excitement

- Keep repeating mistakes

- Personal and organizational stagnation

ACTIVITY 5-5

MINDMAPPING
1. Create a mindmap of Chapter 5 in your textbook.
2. Brainstorm a list of ways to cope with great amounts of change in rapid succession in the healthcare field using the mindmapping technique.

REFERENCE

Rogers, E. (1983). Diffusion of Innovations, 3rd ed., 223–238. New York: Free Press.

CHAPTER 6

PROBLEM SOLVING AND DECISION MAKING

Joseph B. Hurst, Ph.D., Ed.D., and Mary J. Keenan, Ph.D., R.N.

INTRODUCTION

Many people tend to think of the processes of problem solving and decision making as being the same. This chapter clarifies the distinctions between them and discusses how to increase your skills in solving problems and making decisions. Harrison (1981) outlined a basic managerial process for decision making: set objectives, search for options, evaluate options, choose, implement, and follow up/control. Notice that this is similar to the problem-solving process without the focus upfront on problem definition.

OBJECTIVES

- To increase your skills in problem solving and decision making.

- To increase your skills in assisting others in their problem solving and decision making.

ACTIVITY 6-1

Read Chapter 6 in the textbook. Pick a real problem or decision and use the processes described in the text (or another process you or the instructor chooses) to solve your problem, or make your decision. Write out (or create a mindmap of) what you do at each stage (e.g., define problem: "From the staff's perspective, the real problem seems to be... while from the patients' view it appears to be..."). Notice how this structure is similar to and different from how you normally solve problems or make decisions.

Notice how much you relied on yourself to solve the problem or make the decision. Why?

ACTIVITY 6-2

Use the problem definition, force-field analysis, and gap analysis forms that follow on pages 50 through 55 in this workbook to define and analyze a real problem you face. Write out (or map) each of those ways of looking at your problem. What do you notice about your problem now?

What changes in how you might solve it come to mind, including who and what could assist you in solving this problem?

ACTIVITY 6-3

PROBLEM DEFINITION

There are many different ways to define a problem, starting with the way that you and I see it. One way is ask and answer the four questions below. Select a problem, select a partner, and follow through with the questions below.

1. Who and what is affected in what "problematic ways"?

   Who (as I see it):

   Who (as you see it):

   What (as I see it):

   What (as you see it):

2. Who and/or what is causing it?

   Who (as I see it):

   Who (as you see it):

   What (as I see it):

   What (as you see it):

3. What type of a problem is being confronted?

   The problem (as I see it):

   The problem (as you see it):

4. What are the intended goals/specific results to remedy the situation?

   Specific goal, results (as I see it):

   Specific goal, results (as you see it):

Using these four guidelines requires other considerations related to each element of the problem definition. As you formulate and write problem definitions, you can reflect about the following:

1. Who and/or what is affected in what problematic ways? Consider these possibilities: How many people, and who specifically, are negatively affected? What other things are affected and how?

2. Who and/or what is causing this problem? What people are causing this problem, especially in the ways they are interpreting the circumstances and what is happening?

3. What type of problem is being confronted? What is this problem really about: Is it missing resources; a lack of training/skills; power struggles; inaccurate, inadequate, or superfluous communication; a lack of clarity of mission, priorities, roles, and/or norms; poor performance and/or results; misunderstandings; unethical actions; poor public relations, etc.?

Is this really a conflict over information, goals, means, or values/standards rather than a problem to solve? Is it a dilemma that has been mismanaged, or treated like a solvable problem?

4. What are the specific goal(s) and intended result(s) to remedy this situation? Goals:

Intended results:

How would the situation look if this problem was completely solved? What will be the same and what will be different?

(Adapted from Jung, Pino, & Emory, 1973.)

ACTIVITY 6-4

FORCE-FIELD ANALYSIS

Another way to define, analyze, and break problems into smaller ones is to determine the factors (people, time, resources, conditions, procedures, norms, information, relationships, rules, etc.) that block a desired/intended future state and those that support attaining it. Given a problem statement like the one above, a force-field analysis is a listing and realistic weighing of the present and predictable factors that are blocks/barriers to and supports for obtaining the intended future. After deciding on a problem you are presently trying to solve, do the following:

1. Write out a problem statement of the situation.

2. Make a list of the blocking and supporting factors using the force-field analysis form on page 59 of this workbook.

3. Star (or rank order) those that have the most weight.

4. Determine whether the blocking or supporting forces are strongest. Identify subproblems or key focal points by noting major blocks to overcome and major supports to use.

5. Use two or more of the problem-solving techniques discussed in the text (e.g., brainstorming, decision grids, payoff tables, decision trees, PERT charts) to work toward a solution to it.

6. Involve other people in your problem solving.

FORCE-FIELD ANALYSIS FORM

Blocking Forces   **Supportive Forces**

Key Subproblems/Focal Points to Deal With Immediately

ACTIVITY 6-5

GAP ANALYSIS

A gap analysis is another way of envisioning problem solving.

Description of Present Undesired State and Conditions	Description of Desired Future State/Conditions

FORCE-FIELD ANALYSIS

Blocking Factors/Forces	Supporting Factors/Forces

GAP ANALYSIS FORM

PROBLEM AREA(S)

PRESENT STATE OF AFFAIRS   DESIRED STATE OF AFFAIRS

___

ACTIVITY 6-6

1. Discuss the different problems students are having regarding learning this material, completing assignments, and/or doing clinical practice/work. List (and/or map) as many different statements as you can as long as they refer to actual difficulties concerning decision making, problem solving, and learning. Form small groups of volunteers to work on one of the problems together.

2. Define the problem and identify several options to solving it.

   The problem:

   Solutions:
   a)

   b)

   c)

   Draw a diagram of a decision tree of consequences for three of the options and decide on which options to choose.

   Consequences:
   a)

   b)

3. Briefly analyze your problem solving to this point. After class, set up ways to take action and report back at some later date to the entire group.

   Actions:
   a)

   b)

   c)

ACTIVITY 6-7

1. Form a group of four or five students and discuss real problems related to this class or your entire schedule of classes, your practical or work experience, and your experiences in learning to solve problems and make decisions more effectively. Decide on one problem to use as a way of demonstrating the application of your knowledge in this chapter.
2. Request input from the class for a problem definition, gap analysis, and force-field analysis. As the instructor writes these on a chart pad or blackboard, listen and share what you think would add to the process.

ACTIVITY 6-8

MINDMAPPING

1. Create a mindmap of Chapter 6 in your textbook.
2. Use mindmapping to brainstorm alternatives to solve the problem chosen for Activity 6-7, including its associated subproblems, and to decide how individuals and groups in the class can take action and evaluate results. Report back to the class. Write the problem in the middle of a large sheet of paper or poster board. Then map its desired results, action steps, needed resources, barriers, support people available, and timeline.

REFERENCE

Harrison, E. (1981). The managerial decision making process. Boston: Houghton Mifflin.

Jung, C., Pino, R., & Emory, R. (1973). RUPS: Research Using Problem Solving (Leaders Manual). Portland, OR: Northwest Regional Laboratory.

PART 2

MANAGING THE ORGANIZATION

CHAPTER 7

HEALTHCARE ORGANIZATIONS

Mary J. Keenan, Ph.D., R.N., and Marsha Brown, M.S.N., R.N.

INTRODUCTION

Changes in the healthcare system, its organizations, and its financing are bringing about rapid developments in the modes and sites of care delivery. As acute care facilities become more focused on the acutely ill, community facilities that focus on people who are less acutely ill are being developed. No longer are people who are ill or who need surgery cared for in acute hospitals. They are in intermediate care agencies, clinics, and at home. This chapter focuses on how the community is changing its healthcare facilities, changes in healthcare delivery that have occurred in the past five years, and the emerging trends.

OBJECTIVES

- To describe the changes and shifts in the patient census in at least two of the agencies in which you have had clinical experience.

- To identify how delivery of nursing care (systems) have changed over the past five years.

- To describe how the role of nurses is changing in response to the demands in the changing healthcare field.

- To predict what will occur in the next five (or three) years in healthcare delivery.

ACTIVITY 7–1

COMMUNITY SCAVENGER HUNT

Form a group with three to five of your classmates who identify themselves as highly committed and productive. Assume that you have been charged with the responsibility to provide the local health planning community with definitive information that they can use for future planning.

1. Scan community publications (e.g., newspapers, magazines, brochures, etc.) to develop a scenario of what the healthcare scene in your community was like five years ago and how it has changed in yearly increments. Write your description of the agencies and services available in the space below:

What healthcare was like 5 years ago:

4 years ago:

3 years ago:

2 years ago:

1 year ago:

Today:

2. Answer the following questions:
   How many new agencies have been established? What are they?

   How have existing ones been modified by adding programs, redesigning facilities for different services, combining with others, etc.?

Describe the patients (clientele) served then and now, using the following questions as guidelines:
How has acuity changed?

How have census and access changed?

How has professional nursing staffing changed?

How have their healthcare demands changed?

How have reimbursement systems (insurance, HMOs, etc.) changed, expanded, declined?

3. Using your answers to the questions in item 2 above, develop a visual representation (such as a form, grid, mindmap, graph, chart, table, etc.) to depict the changes in the agencies.
4. Based on the information you have gathered, what are your conclusions? What trends can you identify?

5. Using the information you have gathered, and keeping in mind the trends you just described, write a scenario that predicts the future. You already have all the data you need to do so. You know as much as anyone!

ACTIVITY 7–2

BUILD A COLLAGE

1. Collect news articles, magazine articles, photos, advertisements, brochures, etc. regarding local healthcare services, or services in some identifiable region. List your article titles below:

2. Organize them into time frames or developmental stages. Highlight new agencies and services within the time period(s) you select.

3. Identify geographic areas with the newest developments and expansions, perhaps with a creative visual or map.

4. On a poster board, create a visual collage that displays the historical trends in healthcare delivery in the area(s) you have selected.

5. Present your collage to the class.

ACTIVITY 7–3

MINDMAPPING

1. Create a mindmap of Chapter 7 in your textbook.
2. Do an extensive mindmap of either, or both, of the first two activities. Be creative, emphasizing the future and trends you have identified.

CHAPTER 8

CULTURAL DIVERSITY

Rosalind M. Peters, M.S.N., R.N.

INTRODUCTION

The purposes of the exercises in this chapter are, first, to help you examine your own cultural attitudes to determine how they influence your behavior, and second, to compare and contrast your cultural beliefs and practices with those of others who come from a different cultural background.

OBJECTIVES

- To define culture.

- To determine the impact that culture has on health beliefs, health practices, and healthcare delivery.

- To analyze personal cultural beliefs and values to determine their impact on your professional practice.

- To determine the impact of spirituality on health practices.

- To examine the health practices of different cultural groups.

- To determine the level of cultural diversity in your workplace.

ACTIVITY 8–1

CULTURAL DIVERSITY EXERCISE: CULTURAL AWARENESS

1. Describe the differences between the terms *culture, race,* and *ethnicity.*

2. List at least six common characteristics usually associated with the middle–class American culture.
   a)
   b)
   c)
   d)
   e)
   f)

3. Describe common characteristics found in the culture of Western scientific medical practice (e.g., belief in medical model, germ theory).

4. Identify the four most prominent cultural groups in your area.
   a)
   b)
   c)
   d)

   Choose two groups for an in-depth study. Identify the groups in relation to their health beliefs/customs in the areas of birth and death, and their use of folk healers or folk medicines.

5. Determine four similarities and four differences between the "folk medicine" and "Western, scientific medicine" systems.

SIMILARITIES	DIFFERENCES
a)	a)
b)	b)
c)	c)
d)	d)

ACTIVITY 8–2

CULTURAL VALUES CHECKLIST

The following is a short checklist regarding culturally determined values, attitudes, and beliefs, especially as they pertain to healthcare. You must choose to strongly agree, agree, disagree, or strongly disagree with each statement as it is written. This requires that you be as introspective as possible to determine where you stand on each of the issues presented. Please remember that there is no right or wrong answer, just individual attitudes and beliefs. By answering as honestly as possible, this exercise will help you be more conscious of your own culturally determined beliefs.

Read each statement carefully, then circle the answer that most closely reflects your beliefs regarding each statement.

SA=Strongly Agree   A=Agree   D=Disagree   SD=Strongly Disagree

1. Only a small percentage of Americans use alternate forms of healing other than traditional medical science.

   SA A D SD

2. People can change the outcome of serious medical conditions with prayer.

   SA A D SD

3. True grief is expressed with loud sobbing and copious crying.

   SA A D SD

4. Life support should be removed from a person who is brain–dead with no possible hope for recovery.

   SA A D SD

5. Patients should be allowed to have family members at their bedside 24 hours a day.

   SA A D SD

6. Family members should donate a deceased person's organs (as appropriate) so others may be helped.

   SA A D SD

7. Good health is largely determined by a person's diet, exercise, and other similar activities.

   SA A D SD

8. It is important for nurses to question a physician if the nurse is unsure of the rationale behind the physician's orders.

   SA A D SD

9. To get a good patient history, it is important for the nurse to write down the information as the patient is speaking to make sure that none of the information is missed.

   SA A D SD

10. Family members should not be allowed to perform support tasks such as bathing the patient while the patient is hospitalized.

    SA A D SD

11. To be an effective communicator, it is important to maintain good eye contact with people.

    SA A D SD

12. If an employee is not performing satisfactorily, it is important for the manager to speak directly to that person, even if it involves giving straightforward criticism.

    SA A D SD

13. Patting an employee on the back or on top of the head is a friendly gesture to say thanks for a job well done.

    SA A D SD

14. Providing psychosocial care is an important part of being a nurse and nurse manager.

    SA A D SD

For each of the 14 statements in the previous checklist, identify one cultural group that would agree and one that would not:

1. AGREE   DISAGREE

2. AGREE   DISAGREE

3. AGREE   DISAGREE

4. AGREE   DISAGREE

5. AGREE   DISAGREE

6. AGREE   DISAGREE

7. AGREE   DISAGREE

8. AGREE   DISAGREE

9. AGREE   DISAGREE

10. AGREE   DISAGREE

11. AGREE   DISAGREE

12. AGREE   DISAGREE

13. AGREE   DISAGREE

14. AGREE   DISAGREE

Meet in groups of three or four students to discuss your responses to this exercise. Determine three areas of commonality and three areas of difference among members of your group.

Commonality:
1.
2.
3.

Difference:
1.
2.
3.

One responsibility of a family is to provide healthcare for its members by helping them stay well and taking care of members who are ill. Health promotion activities and care given during illness vary greatly among families. Each function is very much influenced by the family's cultural orientation. Friedman (1992) describes six stages of family health/illness interaction that greatly influence each individual's response to healthcare. These stages are: health promotion, illness recognition, care seeking, healthcare system, acute response, and adaptation to illness/recovery.

It is important to note that the family will not make contact with the healthcare delivery system until at least the fourth stage of this interaction continuum. Therefore, the family may have engaged in a variety of health activities before they ever have contact with anyone in a professional setting.

The Family Health/Illness Practices Inventory is designed to increase awareness of family and cultural values that shape health and illness practices. It is a tool that can increase self–awareness of the cultural factors that shape your current approach to healthcare. When used as an interview tool, it can increase awareness of other cultural perspectives regarding healthcare.

Complete your own Family Health/Illness Practices Inventory. Try to remember what it was like for you as a child growing up, answer the questions based on what your family did before you became a nurse.

FAMILY HEALTH/ILLNESS PRACTICES INVENTORY

Questions to ask:

1. Health promotion:
   Cite three health promotion/disease prevention activities done by your family.
   a)
   b)
   c)
   Did you consider your parents to be healthy, frail, sickly? What about your siblings?
   How did your family define *health*?

2. Illness recognition:
   Who was the primary person in the family responsible for determining if a family member was ill?
   Who was primarily responsible for determining what should be done about the illness?
   Who in the family was seen as the "health expert"?

3. Care seeking:
   Who did the family turn to for information regarding the illness if the family was unable to resolve the problem on its own?
   Did the family discuss the problems with extended family members, neighbors, or friends, or go straight to a health professional?

4. Healthcare system:
Did the family use folk practitioner/healers?
Where was the initial contact with the healthcare delivery system made (e.g., healer, private physician, clinic, hospital)?
Who in the family was responsible for deciding where to seek help?

5. Acute response:
What did it mean to be "sick" in your family?
What behaviors were expected of the sick person and of other family members in relation to the sick member?
If it was a serious illness or crisis, how did the family cope with a crisis?
Who was seen as the leader in times of crisis?
What happened if the traditional leader was sick?

6. Adaptation to illness/recovery:
Did anyone in the family have a chronic illness?
How did that affect the other family members?
Who did the family depend on for support (physical, emotional)?

After completing your own Family Health/Illness Practices Inventory, interview someone from a different cultural background. Explain that you are trying to learn more about how different cultures and families view health and illness. Assure the person that the information will be kept confidential. Or seek out a classmate whose cultural background is different from yours and mutually compare and discuss your responses.

ACTIVITY 8–4

SCENARIO

Nancy Jones is a 23-year-old white, middle-class, Protestant nurse who works on the midnight shift of the hospital's oncology unit. Nancy phoned you and asked for your help in solving a patient problem.

When you get to the unit you hear loud moaning and crying coming from the waiting room. You see five men standing in the hallway, talking loudly in a foreign language; you don't know what they are saying, but they seem to be arguing. Walking past the waiting room you notice at least ten other adults and five children. Most of the women are crying. You also notice an unusual odor and find that two women are using the utility room microwave and preparing what looks like a soup.

The patient is B.T., a 29-year-old man who recently immigrated to the United States. He was admitted from the emergency room, diagnosed with acute appendicitis. Blood work and further evaluation revealed an acute leukemic crisis with leukemic infiltrates to the lungs and brain. He is unconscious and has been spiking high fevers. The family reported that B.T. has been fighting a "cold" for the past couple of weeks but they brought him to the hospital because of severe abdominal pain. He has not been under a physician's care and there is no history of leukemia. Because of the seriousness of his condition, medical treatment must begin immediately. Surgery will probably be required for the appendicitis, but the hematologist will need to be involved in that decision also.

Nancy further reports that since B.T. was admitted to the unit more family members have been arriving. Originally, he was accompanied by his wife, an uncle, and two children. As each member arrived, the noise level increased. Nancy asked them to stay in the waiting room, because they don't all speak English, Nancy finds it difficult to communicate with them and they have been pacing between the patient's room and the waiting room.

Nancy also reported that the uncle refuses to leave the patient alone with her and watches her every action "like a hawk." He did not want Nancy to give B.T. a sponge bath to bring the fever down as he wanted to do personal care activities himself. The uncle has barred the wife from coming into the patient's room and states that she is not to be consulted regarding any medical decisions. The uncle, as head of the family here in the United States, viewed himself as responsible for B.T., making all the appropriate decisions, and telling B.T.'s wife what she needs to know. Nancy is in a quandary as she needs a consent form signed for a bone marrow procedure and the uncle doesn't want her to discuss it with the wife. Nancy further reports that she thinks the "soup" is intended for the patient, but she hasn't a clear answer on that.

As you are talking with Nancy, Shirley Smith, M.D., the oncology resident, approaches you. She is furious, stating that the uncle has refused to allow her to examine B.T. and "ordered" her to get a "real" doctor (meaning a man). Nancy and Shirley then start to complain about the "macho arrogance" of the uncle. They also complain about all the other relatives who are making too much noise and disturbing the night for the rest of the patients on the unit. Shirley says she thinks they ought to call security and ask them to "get rid of the whole bunch of them" so that they can get some work done.

Write a brief paragraph describing the steps that you would take in this situation. Use the following questions to guide your writing.

1. What is your initial reaction to the patient/family as described?

2. What is your initial reaction to Nancy and Shirley's suggestion to ask security to remove the family members?

3. How similar are your personal cultural values to the ones described in this family situation?

4. How will you manage the following issues?

   a) obtaining necessary consents

   b) determining who needs to know and understand about the diagnosis and treatment for this patient

   c) providing quiet for the other patients on the unit

   d) respecting the family's desire to be with the patient

   e) respecting the family's desire to have the uncle do some aspects of the patient's personal care

   f) determining why the soup is being made and what to do if it is intended for the patient

   g) supporting the family to accept a female physician

5. How would you advise Nancy and Shirley to cope with this situation?

The purpose of this exercise is to explore the impact of cultural diversity in a work setting. It is designed to identify areas of cultural conflict and to discover how to help resolve similar conflicts in your own workplace.

Form groups of five to seven students. Select who will role play each of the three roles described below (John Smith, Lomar, and Zerena), and who will be observers.

PART I: ROLES

Head Nurse/Observers

As you watch the role play, identify areas of cultural conflict. Determine why you think the conflict is occurring and then determine a plan to resolve the problems that you have identified. Take notes about the verbal and nonverbal responses of each of the participants. Following the role play, discuss how the head nurse could manage the situation presented.

Role Players: John Smith, Lomar, and Zerena.

Read role descriptions, and build upon these to amplify and portray the person that you are representing.

Following the role play discuss three areas of commonality and three areas of difference among the players

Commonality:

1)

2)

3)

Difference:

1)

2)

3)

Both of the new staff nurses, Lomar and Zerena, have very recently arrived in the United States from their homelands. Each has worked as a nurse for many years in hospitals that provide care in a manner very similar to the ones used in this hospital. Both can speak "textbook" English, but are unsure of many of our slang sayings.

PART II: ROLE DESCRIPTIONS

Preceptor, John Smith: You have been a charge nurse on this unit for many years and the head nurse depends on you in many different ways. Today, you have been asked to act as a preceptor to two new foreign nurses who will be joining your unit. Your responsibility is to introduce the two new staff members to each other. Ask them to say a few words to each other about themselves. Then you take them on a tour of your unit (walk around the room and describe different parts of what would be on the unit). At the end of the tour, you tell the new nurses to get lunch while you speak to the head nurse. After the new nurses leave, you turn to the head nurse/observers and start complaining about them, how they talk or are silent, about how they maintain or do not maintain eye contact, about the five different amulets and charms one was wearing, about the "smells of some strong herbs" coming from one of them.

Lomar: You are from a country where being polite and respectful is of the utmost importance. You will never interrupt another person, never contradict them, never tell them straightforwardly if you find their behavior offensive. You are extremely quiet, speaking only when spoken to and even then you will often respond only nonverbally, such as with a shrug or nod of the head. If you must speak, you do so in a very hushed, subdued tone and you never make eye contact because that is considered to be very rude. It is not polite in your country to ask questions, especially of a man. It is also impolite to stand less than three feet away from another person. When asked to say a few words about yourself, you discuss professional information only; it would be impolite to give any personal information at this first meeting. When you are on the tour, you will stay three to four feet behind the others. You walk with your head down and your eyes downcast.

Zerena: You are from a country where people are expected to be very expressive. This means talking loud and gesturing with your arms. Whenever anyone talks to you, you stand very close to them, (about one foot away) while you hold the arm or in some way touch the person you are speaking with. To be polite, you stare very intently at whomever is talking to show your interest. When asked to say a few words about yourself, you offer profuse information including personal information. You constantly ask questions, often interrupting the preceptor as this is an acceptable way to show your interest and attention.

QUESTIONS FOR DISCUSSION

1. What were your initial reactions to Lomar and Zerena?
   Lomar
   Zerena
2. Which of these nurses would you most like to have work on your unit?
   Why?

3. Why would you not want to work with the other nurse?

4. Cite two areas of conflict you would expect might occur on the unit with these two new nurses.
   a)

   b)

5. As a manager, how would you manage John's complaints? Cite two ways.
   a)
   b)
6. Cite two steps you would take to resolve the potential conflicts that you identified in question 4.
   a)
   b)
7. Could/should you have managed this initial meeting any differently? How?

ACTIVITY 8–6

MINDMAPPING

Draw a mindmap that depicts the major concepts presented in Chapter 8. Include effects of culture on health beliefs, heath practices, and healthcare delivery. Identify and include specific actions you can take to incorporate these effects into nursing services to benefit patients, families, and personnel.

REFERENCE

Friedman, M. (1992). Family Nursing: Theory and Practice, 3rd ed., 6–8. Norwalk, CT: Appleton & Lange.

CHAPTER 9

ORGANIZATIONAL STRUCTURE AND THEORY

Marcy R. Bugajski, B.S.N., R.N., and Paula Bonell, B.S.N., R.N.

INTRODUCTION

This chapter discusses organizational structures, mission, goals, vision, and culture. It is designed to assist you to recognize how the values and vision of the overall organization are stated, published, and fulfilled throughout all units, including the nursing units. Together, with the addition of beliefs and values the expressed philosophy and mission make up the foundation for an organization's identity, both present and future.

This chapter determines how your responsibilities and role functions as a nurse would vary in different organizational structures.

OBJECTIVES

* **To compare and contrast three types of organizational structure.**

* **To analyze how vision and mission are related to shared governance.**

* **To analyze the aspects of organizational culture and how they affect an organization.**

ACTIVITY 9-1

You have just moved and are seeking employment at Woodland Hospital. You have reviewed Chapter 9 in the textbook prior to meeting with the nurse recruiter. After reading the mission and vision statement, you decide that this would be your choice for employment, as the hospital espouses shared governance. In discussing how shared governance is in place at this institution, you identify that your role will include the specific responsibilities listed below. Write a one to two sentence response for each statement.

1. Quality improvement unit projects would require your active participation in the following ways:

   a)

   b)

   c)

2. List some interactions/communications you might use with your nursing peers and other health professionals in regard to:

   a) decision making:

   b) formulating unit goals:

   c) questioning unit policies:

   d) power sharing:

The new chief nursing officer for the Cady Institute is reviewing several theories and philosophies in preparation for implementing one that can carry the organization into the next century. In perusing the literature, it became apparent that the concept of shared governance was most appealing for it seemed consistent with the mission of the institution as well as that of the nursing division. You have been appointed to the new committee that has been formed to review the requirements to be considered prior to this change. As a responsible member of this committee deliberating the proposed change, you have been requested to review the literature and cite at least three advantages and three disadvantages for this proposal.

Advantages of shared governance:
1.

2.

3.

Disadvantages of shared governance:
1.

2.

3.

Having completed this assignment, you report your findings to the committee at large. The committee then requests you to compare shared governance to participatory management and formulate a response supporting either management style.

You respond, "I have listed the pros and cons of each type of governance for your consideration prior to recommending adoption of one or the other."

Participatory management has the following advantages:
1

2.

3.

Participatory management has the following disadvantages:
1.

2.

3.

The reasons you give reflect that you have also compared the advantages and disadvantages of participatory management.

YOUR RECOMMENDATION:

I recommend that (select one) be adopted for the following reasons:

Your recommendation was based on the following considerations (please describe each in one or two sentences):

1. How does the educational level of staff affect the decision?

2. What style(s) of managerial leadership are preferred?

3. How are nursing staff members demonstrating autonomy?

ACTIVITY 9-3

As the administrative director for the hospice center of Woodland Health-care Center, you have been asked to develop new unit-based mission and vision statements. The organization's existing mission and vision statements are as follows:

MISSION STATEMENT

The mission of Woodland Healthcare Center is to positively affect the health of the community that it serves and to promote the community value of the not-for-profit healthcare delivery system.

VISION STATEMENT

Woodland Healthcare Center will be a leader in providing holistic, comprehensive, and outstanding healthcare services to the people of this community. We will be dedicated to delivering compassionate, respectful, supportive, convenient, and accessible services to patients and families through an integrated, multidisciplinary team approach. As ancillary personnel, nurses, physicians, and volunteers, we will be committed to professional and organizational excellence across the healthcare spectrum.

Either form a group of three to five students or do this activity yourself. Consider the following:

a) Who should be requested to contribute to the creation of the new hospice unit mission and vision statements?

b) What would be the desired mix of people and how many of each group would you include and why?

c) What characteristics of the unit environment should be examined prior to developing the statements? Space? Color? Furniture? Visitor accommodations? Other?

d) Develop a three-sentence mission statement for the hospice unit of Woodlawn.

ACTIVITY 9-4

Using the same scenario as in Activity 9-3, consider how, as the unit leader, you might successfully increase the staff's awareness of the unit's mission and vision statements. Is it important that each member of the staff internalize the values stated within each? Why or why not?

Give at least two examples of how the mission statement of the organization and the unit in which you are having clinical experience is expressed in the policies, procedures, and/or climate.

1.

2.

ACTIVITY 9-5

1. Create a mindmap of Chapter 9 in your textbook.
2. Create a mindmap showing how to increase staff awareness about any new policy, procedure, program, equipment, or the like.

PART 3

MANAGING
RESOURCES

CHAPTER 10

MANAGING QUALITY AND RISK

Bonnie Nelson, M.S.N., R.N.

INTRODUCTION

Planning is necessary to improve quality and decrease risk. Total quality management (TQM) and Continuous quality improvement (CQI) programs will help to improve the quality of care that is provided in an institution. Planning is an essential part of these programs and the planning time is well spent. The occurrence of incidents may be costly for the institution. Decreasing those risks will decrease costs and improve the quality of care you provide and improve client satisfaction.

OBJECTIVES

- To identify the process of quality improvement that is occurring in an institution.

- To utilize the process of CQI to identify and change an area that needs improvement in a work environment.

- To identify your customers and their needs.

- To define risk management and investigate how it is done in an institution.

ACTIVITY 10–1

1. Form groups of four in which each group member will conduct his or her own interview with a healthcare professional regarding quality improvement. Select interviewees from the institutions in which you work or have clinical experience or have taken nursing classes. Ask the interviewees to address quality improvement in their institution. You will want to interview people at different levels of the organization to gain a broad perspective of everyone's understanding of the process. Suggested people to interview include the head nurse, staff nurse, unit secretary, physician, director of quality improvement, people from other departments, etc.

2. After interviewing these people, reflect on and answer the following questions:

   a) Did each person give you a similar picture of the quality improvement process? Why or why not?

   b) If there were differences, were they significantly different? Why or why not? (If the differences are significant they can have an impact on how well the quality improvement process works.)

   c) Discuss the interviews in your groups and determine what similarities and differences you found.

If the institution used as the subject in Activity 10–1 has a TQM/CQI plan, obtain a copy of the flowchart for the plan. Compare this institution's plan with the eight steps of quality improvement listed on page 193 in the text. Are there more or fewer steps to your plan? Does your plan meet the needs of the institution or does it need to be changed? Why or why not?

ACTIVITY 10–3

Using the eight steps for quality improvement listed in the text, identify one area for improvement and work through the eight steps. In the space below, write out a short progress report about what you accomplished.

Obtaining information from your customers is very important when assessing quality of care. Interview five clients regarding quality of care. The following are some suggested questions to use in your interview:

1. What was most satisfying about the care you have received?

2. What was least satisfying about the care you have received?

3. Have there been any delays in the care that was provided (pain medication delayed, meal tray served late, call light not answered)?

4. Who was most attentive to your specific needs (physician, nurse, nursing assistant, housekeeper)?

5. What would you like to see changed?

6. What would you like to see stay the same?

7. Would you recommend this institution to others?

8. Is there anything else you would like to share regarding the quality of care you have received?

ACTIVITY 10–5

Obtain a copy of the form used in an institution to report incidents or occurrences. Interview a nurse manager or staff nurse regarding the following:

1. What happens to the occurrence report after it is filled out?

2. What types of incidents are to be reported?

3. What is the most frequently occurring incident?

4. How is corrective action taken after an occurrence has taken place?

MINDMAPPING

1. Create a mindmap of Chapter 10 in your textbook.
2. Your text has suggested that you list every person with whom you interact for one week. Do this by mindmapping, identifying your internal and external customers. In addition, interview others about whom they view as their customers. Did they include some that were different from yours?

CHAPTER 11

MANAGING TIME AND PLANNING EFFECTIVE MEETINGS

Joseph B. Hurst, Ph.D., Ed.D.

INTRODUCTION

Do you feel stressed, unproductive, and/or disorganized about all you have to accomplish? Are you frustrated by a lack of time for your priorities? Do you have a sense that you seem to be wasting a lot of time? Do you need some time for yourself? If you answered "yes" to these questions, then this chapter can help by showing you that the solution is not to manage time but to manage your priorities, accomplishments (task completions and results), and energy/commitment. By focusing on time-saving techniques, you can treat the symptoms of disorganization and fluctuating commitment. Activities 11–1 through 11–3 focus on how to identify your priorities in life, plan effectively to accomplish them, acknowledge those accomplishments, and energize yourself for continued action. The key is to shift *from* using your memory and/or daily "to-do" lists to manage your priorities and energy *to* developing a weekly planning system that identifies and acknowledges your priority accomplishments on a regular basis.

Activities 11–4 through 11–6 are designed to familiarize you with several ways to organize, conduct, participate in, and follow up on meetings. It has been said that meetings are a place where you can go to take "minutes" on what you have "wasted hours" to do. These activities will help you learn to use meeting time more efficiently and avoid some common pitfalls.

OBJECTIVES

- To assess your present ways of planning and either adapt them or create new ones to increase your level of organization and sense of accomplishment, decrease your stress level, and increase your energy and commitment.

- To assess how time is wasted in your clinical or work setting and to identify ways to reduce or eliminate them.

- To assess the strengths and weaknesses of meetings in which you participate.

- To develop effective agendas for meetings.

- To examine and adapt an orderly set of procedures for setting up, conducting, and following up on meetings.

- To practice roles needed to conduct effective meetings and to determine how you can increase the effectiveness of your meeting leadership and membership.

ACTIVITY 11–1

1. Read pages 208 to 209 in the textbook. Notice that there are several activities aimed at developing statements of your priority goals and actions to reach them.

2. Complete Exercise 11-1 on text page 208 in writing and read your responses to someone who knows you well. Ask the person to listen to your goals and prioritize to assist you in making them specific and clear. Request the person's support in working toward these priorities.

ACTIVITY 11–2

Examine the prevention and control strategies and tools (text pages 210 to 215) for time management (e.g., priority grid, time log, shift flow sheet, client data card).

How can these strategies and tools (and others you create or find) assist you to implement your plans to reach your priorities?

How will you note and acknowledge your accomplishments?

ACTIVITY 11–3

Create a personal system, or adapt your present one, to include the following:

1. Visual symbolic and written records (perhaps in a creative mindmapped form!) of your short- and long-term priorities including a mission statement and ways to decrease your biggest time wasters (see text Chapter 11).

2. Specific listings of important actions to be completed (taking them out of your memory and committing them to paper) on a weekly basis.

3. Some rating system to note the completion of those activities and goals including (a) accomplished, (b) moved to another time, (c) delegated to someone else, and (d) deleted due to a change in priority.

4. Using the rating system as a record of your accomplishment of your priorities, which is much different than a "to-do" list.

5. As Covey (1989) suggests in *The Seven Habits of Highly Effective People*, write down (or create a mindmap for) your key roles (e.g., supervisor at work, choir director at church, parent, self) and two or three goals/actions you intend to complete in the next week for each role (including weekly organizing on a day convenient for you!), and proactively live your plan with self discipline.

6. Try out and revise your system until you have one that works for you, even if it is your own personal way of using something that you purchase. (The main point here is to create and adapt ways to do this in the future as your commitments, priorities, and lifestyle change.) Use the items below and the rating system to assess your progress and the positive results of your acknowledgment system.

RATING STATEMENTS

I am doing more of the following (1 = not at all to 5 = frequently):

____ 1. identifying my priorities in writing

____ 2. acknowledging what I am getting completed

____ 3. transferring, delegating, and deleting what I do not get done

____ 4. focusing on priorities and completions rather than incompletions and lower priorities

____ 5. planning on a weekly basis

I am experiencing increases (1 = small to 5 = large) in:

____ 1. organization

____ 2. sense of accomplishment

____ 3. energy

____ 4. completed tasks and productivity

____ 5. efficiency

____ 6. confidence

____ 7. sense of competence/power

I am experiencing decreases (1 = small to 5 = large) in:

____ 1. wasted time

____ 2. incomplete tasks

____ 3. feeling stressed and overwhelmed

____ 4. procrastination

____ 5. forgotten commitments

How could you adapt and use your personal "acknowledgment system" in the future to maintain or increase these results?

ACTIVITY 11–4

Examine the diagram on how to structure a meeting's agenda on page 103 of this workbook. Notice how a meeting can be divided into three different sections (1) info sharing—minutes, announcements, news flashes; (2) decisions and conversations for action; and (3) items for further discussion and group processing. Given the list of agenda items below, organize a two-hour meeting to address them all. Use the above structure to order these items. List them in an agenda with specific time limits for each item.

AGENDA ITEMS

a. 10 minutes to discuss how to make team meetings more effective
b. 30 minutes to decide on a new schedule format
c. 10 minutes to share news
d. 20 minutes to discuss new possibilities for continuous improvement on the unit
e. 5 minutes to decide when to hold shift party
f. 10 minutes to review last meeting's minutes
g. 10 minutes to revise report form
h. 5 minutes to discuss items for the next meeting
i. 10 minutes to give out assignments
j. 10 minutes to answer questions

MEETING AGENDA STRUCTURE

INFORMING: EXCHANGING

F
I
R   •   **Introductions**
S
T   •   **Checking Minutes**

   •   **Announcements**

T
H   •   **Providing Information**
I
R   •   **Obtaining Input From Members**
D
   •   **Making Simple Decisions**

DECISION MAKING: ACTING

M
I   •   **Discussing Options and Consequences (Pros/Cons)**
D
D   •   **Making Decisions (Easy: Difficult: Easy)**
L
E   •   **Organizing/Scheduling Action**

T
H
I
R
D

DISCUSSING: INTERACTING

L
A   •   **For Discussion Items Only**
S
T   •   **Starting a Discussion About Action Needed at a Later Meeting**

   •   **Making Simple Decisions**

T
H   •   **Asking for Questions, Comments, Input, etc.**
I
R   •   **Discussing the Strengths, Weaknesses, and Suggested**
D   **Improvements of the Group's Functioning**

ACTIVITY 11–5

Examine the meeting checklists on pages 105 and 106 of this workbook. Focus your attention on how to structure, prepare for, conduct, and follow up on a meeting.

1. Use these checklists to select one meeting that you have attended recently and rated as "excellent." If you didn't set it up or conduct it, talk to the people who did. Tell them you are studying meetings and would like to learn how the meeting was organized, conducted, and followed up on. Listen and take notes.

2. Compare and contrast how the meeting was planned and run with the checklist items. Then in the space below write a short description of how the meeting may have been more effective from start to finish.

3. Revise or adapt the items to create your own personal checklist for one type of meeting you have regularly in your clinical or work setting. Make sure the structure would fit your meeting's purposes and unit conditions.

4. Use your personal checklist to set up an actual meeting, or in the space below write out a short scenario of how you would set up, conduct, and follow up on your next meeting, as if you were responsible.

MEETING CHECKLIST 1

Planning the meeting

_____1. Determined that the meeting is absolutely necessary; memos, letters, informational "handouts," phone calls, tele-conferences, and/or face-to-face, one-on-one meetings are not more effective.

_____2. Stated the purposes of the meeting concretely.

_____3. Established an agenda including:

___a. Clear purposes stated.

___b. Input from group up until halfway point between meetings (e.g., before second week for monthly meetings).

___c. Time limit set with exact start and stop times.

___d. The meeting schedule is printed with background material attached. Schedule is planned using the $\frac{1}{3}$ principle.

___e. First $\frac{1}{3}$ of meeting time used for easy items including short ice-breaker, approval of minutes/summary, quick action and commitment.

___f. Middle $\frac{1}{3}$ for discussion and commitment to action with hardest item last within this third of meeting.

___g. Last $\frac{1}{3}$ for discussion only (e.g., possibilities, brainstorming, issues to be resolved) with hardest item first and easiest last.

_____4. Typed, revised, printed and sent out agenda so it arrived on day $\frac{3}{4}$ of time between meetings (e.g., at end of third week for a monthly meeting).

_____5. Arranged for people to take minutes and support summary completion.

_____6. Established and communicated long-range schedule of meetings.

_____7. Delegated the tasks for handling all room arrangements, including materials, speaker, handouts, etc.

___a. Room is scheduled.

___b. Room is neat, organized, lighted, correct temperature, etc.

___c. Equipment is there in working operation.

___d. Important speakers are reminded and prepared.

___e. Delegatees promise to complete tasks and report completion.

_____8. Check off all items on planning checklist including any items added below.

_____

_____

_____

_____

MEETING CHECKLIST 2

Running the meeting

____1. Started exactly on time.

____2. Kept to the agenda, covering all items and not introducing new items. (Called "emergency meeting" to handle unexpected, high priority items.)

____3. Called on people for input, feedback, etc.

____4. Drew out quiet members.

____5. Requested vocal members allow others to speak.

____6. Requested that arguments, personal criticisms, etc. be handled outside the meeting and set a time for this to be scheduled and completed.

____7. Kept agenda activities on schedule; respected meeting purpose(s).

____8. Asked for clarification of terms, points, etc., and/or paraphrased them for clarification.

____9. Listened and spoke so that commitment to action, accountability, deadline dates, etc., were clear and written down.

____10. Led through political and intellectual discussions and disagreements so possibility, action, and commitment emerged (e.g., assignments, between meeting subgroups, scheduling agenda items).

____11. Presided as a personable, neutral moderator.

____12. Brought discussion to a close within time frame.

____13. Shared appreciation for member input, "homework," contributions, etc.

____14. Declared the meeting officially complete.

After the meeting

____1. Shared appreciation.

____2. Scheduled and completed conversations about arguments, criticism, etc.

____3. Followed up on reports, promises, agenda items for next meeting, etc.

____4. Produced and distributed minutes, summary, next meeting's agenda, informational handouts, etc.

____5. Began use of planning checklist #1 for next meeting.

ACTIVITY 11–6

During meetings people need to "play" at least four important roles: facilitator/gatekeeper, recorder/minute taker, timekeeper/agenda moderator, and process observer. See the descriptions of these roles in the box below.

1. Reflect on your participation in past meetings.

2. How have you assisted the group by playing any of these roles?

3. Effective groups rotate these roles so that everyone does them sooner or later. Who tends to play these roles in your meetings and why?

4. How do you think assigning these roles to participants in your regular meetings would affect their productivity? Why?

KEY GROUP/MEETING ROLES TO ASSIGN/VOLUNTEER FOR

Facilitator: Neutrally keeps meeting going and "gatekeeps"–involves people.

Time Keeper: Keeps agenda to time schedule.

Recorder: Writes down key decisions, promises, requests, ideas, etc.

Process Observer: Provides feedback about what is working, not working, and missing.

ACTIVITY 11–7

MINDMAPPING
1. Create a mindmap of Chapter 11 in your textbook.

REFERENCE

Covey, S. (1989). The Seven Habits of Highly Effective People. NY: Simon & Schuster.

CHAPTER 12

MANAGING INFORMATION AND TECHNOLOGY

Rosemary Kahle, M.Ed., R.N., and Bonnie Nelson, M.S.N., R.N.

INTRODUCTION

The computer is such an integral part of our lives that to understand how to use one is as important as knowing how to use a pencil and paper. Nurses must understand how to use the available technology to expedite data processing and communication in the healthcare system. Computers come in a variety of forms and sizes, ranging from the powerful mainframe computers to the small, handheld notebook. They all operate on the same principle for processing information. Computers also aid in accessing information from databases for literature searches. This chapter acquaints you with some of the applications of communication technology to nursing.

OBJECTIVES

- To complete a computerized search using two different data bases.

- To identify the pros and cons of a computerized nursing system.

- To examine issues of confidentiality for computerized patient record system.

- To identify uses for E-mail.

ACTIVITY 12-1

You are the head nurse and you have been asked to participate in the implementation of a computerized nursing information system in the institution. This is a 30-bed unit with a nursing staff comprised chiefly of RNs and some LPNs. The new system to be instituted includes notebook computers to be used at the bedside for nursing care entries. The staff on your unit have been aware that computers are coming and a change will take place, although they are not aware of exactly what it will be, nor of their exact role in it. You are very excited about the powerful potential this new tool has and you want the staff to share your enthusiasm. The staff have mixed feelings, for some of them have indicated that they believe that they are licensed to "take care of patients," not to "run" a computer. Others are very excited about the opportunity to learn a more efficient way to input patient information. Your job is to introduce the change with the least amount of disruption. How are your going to facilitate the needed change?

Prior to planning to meet with the staff, you decide to outline the positions on both sides, that is, those who like it the way it is (status quo) and those who want to learn the new method of bedside charting (progressive). Some people have a position somewhere in the middle— they are somewhat ready for change and to move forward.

1. Review Chapter 12 in the textbook.
2. Compare two aspects of the dilemma by making a list of behaviors for the status quo orientation group and a list of the behaviors for the progressive orientation group.

STATUS QUO	PROGRESSIVE
BEHAVIORS	
a) stable	a) open minded
b) uniform	b) unblocked
c)	c)
d)	d)
e)	e)
PROS	
a) do not have to change	a) new challenge
b) no disruption with patient care	b) faster data entry
c)	c) instant data retrieval
d)	d)
CONS	
a) present method labor intensive	a) time to learn new system
b) need to have chart to obtain data	b) cost of system
c)	c)
d)	d)

What are the benefits of the progressive orientation?

What are the benefits of the status quo orientation?

What would be the result if only the progressive orientation side is considered?

What are the negatives of the progressive orientation?

What could be the result if only the status quo orientation is considered and the progressive orientation is ignored?

What do people like about both the progressive and the status quo orientation?

ACTIVITY 12-2

COMPUTERIZED LITERATURE SEARCHES

The clinical unit is participating in a clinical research study involving drug addicted infants. It is your task to obtain the latest research documentation regarding nursing care of these infants. The library has two systems for performing literature searches. One method involves using the printed hardbound Cumulative Index to Nursing and Allied Health Literature (CINAHL) series and the other method is accessing the CINAHL data base electronically.

The resources required for the electronic CINAHL search are a computer system with a CD-ROM reader, the CINAHL-CD, and a printer, or a computer that connects to a network, a printer, and the appropriate data base(s).

List three data bases that are available to you at the university library. Cite the capabilities and limitations of each.

Data base
Capabilities

Limitations

Data base
Capabilities

Limitations

Data base
Capabilities

Limitations

1. Are there computers available on which you can perform your own literature search?
2. What are the disadvantages if you cannot access a computer and perform your own searches?

After determining that CINAHL is available at a library to which you have access, and that there is an IBM compatible computer system with a NEC MultiSpin CD-ROM reader and a printer available for student use, search the nursing literature using CINAHL.

1. Obtain the instructions from the librarian for how to access CINAHL. (These instructions will vary from agency to agency.)

2. Every search consists of two major parts, finding the relevant records and showing them on the monitor. If there is a printer available, all or selected records can be printed. A search can also be downloaded to a floppy disk if desired. A search can be conducted by using subject, textword(s), author, name of the journal, or title.

   Approximately 70 percent of the CINAHL subject headings are listed Medical Subject Headings (MeSH) and additionally, there are more than 1,000 headings unique to nursing and allied health. If the search is conducted using textwords, there are Subject Heading Lists available.

3. A search can be performed by entering a single subject word or phrase, such as *nursing* or *critical care*. Using the Boolean operator (words such as *and* and *or*) at the "Find" prompt allows combined search terms and narrows the search. For example, a search combining the terms *nursing* and *critical care* can be entered as *nursing and critical care;* another example is *runaways and health care.*

4. Typing the "in" operator (which simply indicates that you are requesting articles in a certain type of document) by entering the word *in*, with a field label (*dt* = document type) at the "Find" prompt narrows the search and searches the records that meet the specification. If a search is requested to gain only research articles in nursing and critical care, then an entry such as *nursing and critical care and research in dt* will search for records meeting the criteria (nursing and critical care) and all of these records will be research based in the document type.

5. Perform a search. Example: enter *nursing* at the "Find" prompt.

6. View the records on the screen.

7. Select five records for printing.

8. Print the records.

   Questions to consider:
   Is your search manageable or is it too broad?
   If there were too many records were you able to narrow the search?
   Were you able to select the records for printing?
   Were the abstracts (most records have abstracts) part of the printout?

ACTIVITY 12-4

MEDLINE is another data base available to the students in the library. The MEDLINE data base of the U.S. National Library of Medicine contains information from 1966 to the present. Using the MeSH thesaurus, one can search for citations and abstracts in the worldwide biomedical literature. The procedure for searching MEDLINE is very similar to searching CINAHL.

1. Request the instructions for accessing MEDLINE. (These instructions will vary from one agency to another.)

2. Perform a literature search using MEDLINE.

3. The data base is searchable by index terms, author, synonyms, and subject headings (MeSH).

4. Begin the search by entering a single subject word or phrase at the Command Line, such as *diabetes*. Your entry will be automatically searched in the subject fields of the data base.

ACTIVITY 12-5

USING ELECTRONIC MAIL (E-MAIL)

Electronic mail (E-mail) allows people to communicate with each other via computer in a nonintrusive way. It is available if you have a microcomputer that is connected to a network. Just as each person has a home address or a telephone number, so it is with E-mail. You can send mail to anyone, anywhere, providing you know their address.

As the clinical unit manager on ward 8B you need to send a message to the unit manager on ward 4A. In the past you would use the telephone to relay the information, but the phone line might be busy or the person to whom you wish to speak might be unavailable. With E-mail the line is never busy and the person you have the message for need not be available. E-mail is fast and direct and there is no waiting.

The new computer system that was recently installed in the agency is connected to the network and you have been informed that E-mail is available for sending your message to the unit manager on 4A.

1. What is the appropriate address of the recipient?

2. How do you access the E-mail screen?

3. How do you write and send the message?

4. How do you send a message to an institution in another city?

CONFIDENTIALITY

You are the manager on the surgical intensive care unit. All the beds on your unit are full and you are expecting another postoperative patient for admission. You ask the secretary to request a bed on the surgical step-down unit so that a patient may be transferred out of your unit. The secretary pulls up the screen on the computer with the census for the step-down unit and informs you that there is one bed for a woman. You are aware that she has not used the phone to call admitting and you also know that her access code gives her only the census on the unit she is currently working on. You approach her and see the screen on the computer. You ask her how she was able to obtain that screen and she tells you that Dr. Schultz gave her his code so that she would be able to locate beds for his patients more rapidly. But the physician's code could allow the secretary to obtain any information in the computer regarding any patient in the institution, which is unacceptable because of issues of confidentiality.

Consider the following scenarios:

It is important for the admitting office to have control of the appropriate assignment of beds. If the nurse calls the report to the step-down unit in this situation, assuming they have the bed for the ICU patient, and the nurse on the receiving unit accepts the report but does not know that another nurse has already taken the report on a patient in the emergency room for that bed, what are the possible consequences when both patients arrive on the unit at the same time?

Suppose that the ICU patient requires a ventilator and the patient coming from the emergency room is in acute distress. How could this situation have been avoided?

The secretary (who knows Dr. Schultz's access code) has a best friend who has been admitted to the infectious disease unit. Might there be results in the computer that she would like to find out about her friend?

Should she have access to this information? Provide a rationale.

What should you do as the manager when discovering this breach in confidentiality?

What should you do as manager when discovering violation of the security of the computer system?

ACTIVITY 12-7

MINDMAPPING

Working alone or with others, draft a mindmap to portray the advantages, disadvantages, and cautions of computerization within healthcare today and project to tomorrow. Peruse ads in healthcare and hospital journals that suggest current and projected uses for computers. Give free rein to your "futuristic thinking" and to your imagination as you describe today and design tomorrow.

CHAPTER 13

MANAGING COSTS AND BUDGETS

Marsha Brown, M.S.N., R.N., and Mary Ann
Dimmick, M.S.N., R.N.

INTRODUCTION

There are many facets of the budget that we as nurse managers have control over, and there are others for which we have little responsibility. Yet we as managers have a significant role in establishing and monitoring the individual departmental budgets that make up the whole financial picture for the institution. Aside from "guestimating" operating costs for the new fiscal year based on historical data, there is one basic consideration in managing costs and budgets: shrewd management of the departmental full-time equivalents (FTE's). We refer to it as "Scheduling." A thorough understanding of FTE's promotes a cost-effective, cost-efficient, quality care, highly motivated department.

These exercises in this chapter are designed to increase your understanding of the intimate relationships among FTE's, staffing components and ratios, staffing and budgeting, and staffing and patient "case mix."

OBJECTIVES

- **To determine the budgetary effects of overbudgeted hours and overtime.**

- **To develop a minimum staffing schedule for one month.**

- **To calculate relationships and contributions of full-time and part-time personnel in allocating FTE's.**

- **To examine a dilemma that arises from the needs of a patient population and needs of a nursing staff.**

Do this exercise with a partner. Develop charts or other graphic ways to illustrate the following activities.

SCENARIO: EXPANSION!

You have been informed that because of your statistical justification efforts, administration has recognized the need for more monitored beds. This means that your department will expand from its current eleven beds to twenty monitored beds. As a nurse manager, you are initially very pleased about this expansion, but then you feel dismay because you will have a lot of work to do and only a little time in which to accomplish it. You also have an additional 12 FTE's to add to your current 20.5 FTE's. The current staffing mix is as follows:

> RN FTE's = 12 (10 full-time and 4 part-time)
> LPN FTE's = 3.5 (2 full-time and 3 part-time)
> Nursing Assistant FTE's = 1.5 (6 work every other weekend and one works the Friday along with her weekend)
> Nursing Aide FTE's = 1.0 (full-time, works only Monday to Friday)
> Unit Clerk FTE's = 2.5 (2 full-time, work 9 to 5:30 during the week and every other weekend, and 1 part-time, works 6 P.M. to 10 P.M. Monday through Friday)

The additional 12 FTE's include all support personnel (unit clerks, nursing assistants, and aides as well as RNs and LPNs).

Establish the following:

1. List three goals for the new expanded unit. Include patient outcomes such as discharge criteria, acuity level, and patient teaching.

   a)

   b)

   c)

2. Make a list that differentiates the allocation of FTE's of caregivers and support personnel. Some of the support personnel may also be listed as caregivers, such as nursing assistants and/or unit clerks that are cross-trained as nursing aides. Consider the following when doing the allocation.

   a) There are nine more patients who require care.

   b) There are times when there is no unit clerk available and the daytime clerks have to work overtime to cover the period from 5:30 to 6:00 P.M.

   c) Who will be observing nine additional monitors? Would you want to consider a monitor tech or cross-training some of the other available personnel?

   d) Consider patient outcomes — will your patients be on the monitor during their entire stay in the unit and when the monitor is discontinued they are transferred, or will they remain on the unit until discharge and require a lower level of care?

   e) Currently the acuity level is higher than the original staffing plan was designed for, which is resulting in the nursing staff working overtime on a daily basis.

3. Decide how many part-time versus full-time positions you will need to accomplish the goals set forth in #1 above.

Remember that when a part-time person works overtime it is not usually paid at time and a half and they frequently are asked to contribute more to receive benefits.

4. Determine the minimum number of staff necessary for all three shifts. Keep in mind that the staffing ratio on your unit is currently one RN or LPN to four patients. Take into account that full-time staff on your unit currently work twelve-hour shifts and every third weekend.

5. Discuss with your partner and develop a clear rationale to demonstrate your understanding of overbudgeted hours and overtime.

ACTIVITY 13-2

Do this exercise with a partner. Develop your own graphics to demonstrate how you would illustrate this staffing pattern. List the decisions that you must make as you complete this schedule. Supply your rationale for these decisions. Using the scenario and numbers in Activity 13-1, develop a four-week schedule for your department. Keep in mind that you require a minimum staffing ratio of 1:4. Include the following considerations within your schedule:

1. One FTE RN will start maternity leave during the second week of the schedule.

2. A mandatory four-hour safety workshop is scheduled for the second Tuesday of every month from 8 A.M. to 12 Noon. You must send four people this month to meet the quota.

3. There is no scheduled overtime.

4. Three new RNs must attend EKG classes. The classes are scheduled the first three weeks of your four-week schedule on every Wednesday and Thursday from 8 A.M. to 4:30 P.M.

5. One RN is on a medical LOA indefinitely.

6. You have six ACLS instructors on your unit and two of them must attend updates or they will lose their instructor status. The course is scheduled for the third Friday of the month.

7. You will conduct a staff meeting regarding the upcoming changes (day and time of your choice).

8. Nursing grand rounds is scheduled for the last Wednesday of the month from 12 to 1:00 P.M. This is your lucky day. Your unit is presenting and everyone wants to attend.

9. Two unit clerks, one full-time and one part-time, have requested vacation time during the first week of the schedule.

10. There must have been discount airline tickets to Florida this winter. Three RNs have "already purchased tickets" and each is requesting ten days off. Two of them work the same weekend and that weekend is included in the the vacation request.

11. You need an "on-call" list of those willing to work extra when you have those last minute sick call-offs! No overtime is permitted unless you can justify it to administration.

DILEMMA

There are very few, if any, budgetary decisions that are clearly distinct in all components, and once decided upon, never change. This exercise asks you to identify a budgetary dilemma to be managed while meeting the needs of patients and the needs of personnel. Use the space that follows to describe the scenario you have chosen to work with.

Next, follow the suggestions in items 1–4 below to help you gain a balanced understanding of the dilemma that is inherent in budgetary decisions on a nursing unit.

1. Identify two sides of the dilemma, namely, meeting the needs of patients and meeting the needs of personnel.
2. Identify at least five positives for each side.
3. Identify at least five negatives for each side.
4. List at least four suggestions about how to manage this dilemma over time.

Determine an operating budget for personnel in the area where you are currently working. You may use the following guides to assist with this process. Calculate the cost for the personnel.

You will begin by determining the number of staff in each category working in the area. Additional lines are provided for personnel not identified by the example.

Part I Number
#RNs—Full-time, full benefits   _____
#RNs—Part-time, limited benefits   _____
#LPNs—Full-time, full benefits   _____
#LPNs—Part-time, limited benefits   _____
#Nursing assistants/aides,—benefits, if any   _____
#Clerical specialists—Full-time, full benefits   _____
#Clerical specialists—Part-time, limited benefits   _____

_____ _____
_____ _____
_____ _____

Part II
Determine the salary for each group. You may use baseline hourly salaries since figuring cost by years of service becomes very complicated.
RN baseline salary _____
LPN baseline salary _____
Nursing assistant/aide baseline _____
Clerical specialist, baseline salary _____

_____
_____
_____

Add the cost of benefits for each group. For this exercise add 15 percent for benefits for full-time employees and 7.5 percent for part-time employees.
Baseline salary + % baseline = total salary
_____ + _____ = _____ RN full-time
_____ + _____ = _____ RN part-time
_____ + _____ = _____ LPN full-time
_____ + _____ = _____ LPN part-time
_____ + _____ = _____ Nursing assistant/aide if any
_____ + _____ = _____ Clerical specialists full-time
_____ + _____ = _____ Clerical specialists part-time

Part III

Use the following formula to calculate the cost for one month:
Number of staff for category × total salary × hours worked/month = monthly salary .

For example, four full-time RNs × $10/hour × 160 hours = $6,400
Note: base calculations on   full time = 160 hours/month
                               Part time = 80 hours/month

Full-time RNs

_____ × _____ × _____ = _____

Part-time RNs

_____ × _____ × _____ = _____

Full-time LPNs

_____ × _____ × _____ = _____

Part-time LPNs

_____ × _____ × _____ = _____

Nursing assistant/aides

_____ × _____ × _____ = _____

Full-time clerical specialist

_____ × _____ × _____ = _____

Part-time clerical specialists

_____ × _____ × _____ = _____

Other

_____ × _____ × _____ = _____

GRAND TOTAL: _____

MINDMAPPING

Design a blueprint that depicts the interrelationships among 1) staffing, 2) budgeting, and 3) case mix. First examine the components of each of the three components. Next draw a mindmap that depicts the interrelationships among all three components. Draw conclusions as to which (if any) component is more important than the other two. Share you mindmap with others and discuss the implications for your future practice in nursing.

PART 4
LEADING AND MANAGING PEOPLE

CHAPTER 14

TEAM BUILDING

Joseph B. Hurst, Ph.D., Ed.D., Mary J. Keenan, Ph.D., R.N., and Tim Krzys, M.S.N., R.N.

INTRODUCTION

Teamwork is the name of the game these days. In almost every type of institution there is an emphasis on building and maintaining effective teams. Despite this focus on teamwork, many of us still have old habits and beliefs about being effective individuals. Remember all those times you decided, and others encouraged you, to "do it yourself." "Be strong and handle it alone!" Now the game has been changed to cooperating and collaborating. This chapter aims to increase your understanding of what produces high-performing teams, focusing your attention and commitment on a particular task, group-maintaining, and individualistic behaviors and how they affect groups.

OBJECTIVES

- To assess team functioning in groups in which you are a member and recommend ways to improve it.

- To observe member behaviors during team sessions.

- To commit to increased task and maintenance behaviors and reduced individualistic behaviors in group settings.

ACTIVITY 14–1

Read Chapter 14 in the textbook and complete the suggested team assessment for a team you are (or have been) on (pages 278 and 279). Using the scoring guide, select a group of which you have been a member. Using the attributes of effective and ineffective teams in Chapter 14 (page 277), determine how well your group performed on the following four dimensions: objectives, assignments, feelings, and working environment.

ACTIVITY 14–2

1. List at least five criteria for effective teamwork.
   a)

   b)

   c)

   d)

   e)

2. Identify and evaluate three effective measures (what worked) that were used in the group/team you selected for Activity 14-1.
   a)

   b)

   c)

3. Identify and evaluate three ineffective measures.
   a)

   b)

   c)

4. Identify what was missing from the team's performance. Apply criteria to your observations and experience in the group.

5. Based on your reading of Chapter 14 and any other articles, list three specific ways to enrich team performance.
   a)

   b)

   c)

6. Identify and commit to at least two new actions you could take to improve your role as a team member. Write them down and set deadline dates.
   a) I will   by

   b) I will   by

ACTIVITY 14–3

Another way to define effective teamwork is to determine how well members function on the team. In fact, as members contribute the appropriate useful behaviors, they are providing "functional leadership." Such leadership occurs when members engage in behaviors that:

a) contribute to the accomplishment of group tasks and results (task behaviors),

b) contribute to developing and maintaining group cohesion and morale (maintenance behaviors), and

c) avoid selfish tendencies that block group functioning (individualistic behaviors).

Read the description of these behaviors on pages 139 through 143 of the workbook.

1. Cite at least three task, maintenance, and individualistic behaviors you tend to demonstrate presently on at least one team.

a)

b)

c)

2. Cite at least three task and maintenance behaviors you could add (with some stretch and risk) to your typical behaviors, as well as of "replacement" behaviors for any individualistic ones you notice.

a)

b)

c)

OBSERVING AND USING TASK, MAINTENANCE, AND INDIVIDUALISTIC BEHAVIORS

A commonly used method of observing group behaviors is in terms of task, maintenance, and individualistic behaviors. The following sections list a set of task, maintenance, and individualistic behaviors and ways to use them in a group. One approach to viewing positive group membership is to avoid an "underuse" and an "overuse" of each behavior.

Task Behaviors

The behaviors in the chart below help us to get the group started and stimulate the sharing of information, ideas, and opinions. Under each section is a description concerning how the underuse or overuse of a particular type of behavior may affect the group.

TASK BEHAVIORS: STARTING AND SHARING

1. **INITIATORS**: "The first item on our agenda is…"
   a) **Use**: Getting the group started.
   b) **Underuse**: Not initiating when the group needs to get started.
   c) **Overuse**: Initiating when the group needs maintenance or another task direction.

2. **INFORMATION SEEKERS**: "How many people have sent in their registrations?"
   a) **Use**: Increasing data and idea sharing.
   b) **Underuse**: Withholding key questions, letting the group "bog down".
   c) **Overuse**: Seeking more information when enough is available, seeking irrelevant data.

3. **INFORMATION GIVERS**: "Sixty percent of our clients said 'needs improvement'"
   a) **Use**: Providing needed data.
   b) **Underuse**: Not sharing relevant data.
   c) **Overuse**: Supplying irrelevant information, giving biased details, fogging the issue.

4. **OPINION SEEKERS**: "What are our feelings about this idea?"
   a) **Use**: Increasing sharing of opinions, values, and goals.
   b) **Underuse**: Not responding to other's opinions.
   c) **Overuse**: Seeking opinions when facts are needed.

5. **OPINION GIVERS**: "I disagree that it might help us."
   a) **Use**: Letting the group know where members stand on issues.
   b) **Underuse**: Withholding key opinions when needed for group task or maintenance.
   c) **Overuse**: Providing opinions when facts are needed, interjecting irrelevant ideas.

6. **PROCEDURAL FACILITATORS**: "Could we try consensus decision making here?"
   a) **Use**: Helping move group to productive processes of action.
   b) **Underuse**: Resisting change, not moving quickly to new ways of acting.
   c) **Overuse**: Proposing irrelevant or cumbersome procedures.

7. **DOERS:** "I'll be glad to take notes."
   a) **Use:** Completing needed tasks.
   b) **Underuse:** Bogging group down while looking for someone to do the needed actions.
   c) **Overuse:** Trying to do everything at once, doing irrelevant tasks.
8. **RECORDERS:** "Here's what I've written. Is it accurate?"
   a) **Use:** Keeping accurate records of actions taken.
   b) **Underuse:** Losing track of group's past accomplishments, limiting responses when no one volunteers to record or when others view recording as a woman's job.
   c) **Overuse:** Noting irrelevant details, having one person do all the recording.

These task behaviors are important to getting the group started and to sharing needed ideas, opinions, information, and routine tasks. The ones below initiate an even deeper level of problem solving and commitment.

Task Behaviors: Accomplishment and Commitment
1. **ORIENTERS:** "We've been talking about the wealthy for ten minutes. Let's get back to the report."
   a) **Use:** Keeping the group on task.
   b) **Underuse:** Ignoring the task behavior. Keeping the group off task.
   c) **Overuse:** Restricting the group to narrow limits or to one's own way of doing things.

2. **ELABORATORS:** "It sounds like we are talking about product quality instead of...."
   a) **Use:** Providing deeper insights and complexity.
   b) **Underuse:** Maintaining a vague or superficial level when depth is needed.
   c) **Overuse:** Providing depth and complexity too quickly.

3. **COORDINATORS:** "The committee needs to meet tomorrow and share their ideas."
   a) **Use:** Encouraging cooperation and combining of ideas.
   b) **Underuse:** Ignoring the needs for scheduling and planning, and fostering competition.
   c) **Overuse:** Overplanning or building illogical relationships. Planning for others rather than with them.

4. **EVALUATORS:** "So far we have accomplished the following...."
   a) **Use:** Measuring and judging group progress.
   b) **Underuse:** Providing little or no evaluation of group progress.
   c) **Overuse:** Constantly evaluating the group and restricting the freedom to act. Using unrelated standards.

5. **ENERGIZERS:** "I know we can get most of it done in one more hour."
   a) **Use:** Motivating groups to task accomplishments.
   b) **Underuse:** Accepting apathy. Providing little or no motivation.
   c) **Overuse:** Stimulating unproductive activity. Stimulating competition.

These behaviors promote added depth, cooperation, checks on progress, and motivation. Combined with the first eight task behaviors, these actions focus group energy on goal accomplishment and cooperation.

Any member can behave in a variety of task areas during a particular session and over the life of the group. Sometimes all members are involved in one or more of these behaviors (e.g., opinion giving and evaluation) because it is vital to the group's success at that time. These behaviors may involve questions, statements, requests, nonverbal signals, and other behaviors needed for efficient group functioning. One basic question may serve several task functions at the same time (e.g., clarifying, orienting, and opinion seeking). Unfortunately, the same question said in a joking manner might result in individualistic behavior also (e.g., blocking or avoiding).

Maintenance Behaviors

Maintenance behaviors facilitate group process and stimulate positive feelings and interpersonal relationships. Group maintenance is just as important as task behaviors, but is often overlooked by group members. The chart below outlines the effects of the use, underuse, and overuse maintenance behaviors.

1. **ENCOURAGERS**: "I really appreciate your efforts to get this done. Thanks!"
   a) **Use**: Accepting others and showing appreciation for their efforts.
   b) **Underuse**: Discouraging others or failing to encourage them.
   c) **Overuse**: Agreeing dishonestly or superficially

2. **GATEKEEPERS**: "Let's hear from our silent members, what do you think, Steve?"
   a) **Use**: Seeing that communication is open to all members.
   b) **Underuse**: Remaining quiet and allowing others to dominate or remain out of the discussions.
   c) **Overuse**: Dominating communication and controlling other's messages.

3. **HARMONIZERS**: "I'm sure we can find a solution that meets both your criticisms."
   a) **Use**: Relieving tension and build positive relationships.
   b) **Underuse**: Allowing unproductive conflict to continue.
   c) **Overuse**: Avoiding needed conflict or covering over issues with humor and light remarks.

4. **CONFLICT MANAGERS**: "Perhaps we can work out a compromise to resolve this."
   a) **Use**: Helping resolve group disagreements.
   b) **Underuse**: Refusing to compromise, accommodate, cooperate, etc. when needed.
   c) **Overuse**: Competing or yielding when inappropriate.

5. **STANDARD SETTER**: "To help us work together better, let's get to know each other better."
   a) **Use**: Motivating the group toward improved relationships.
   b) **Underuse**: Ignoring interpersonal needs and people's feelings.
   c) **Overuse**: Overemphasizing feelings while avoiding tasks.

6. **WELCOMERS**: "We've missed you. I'm glad you're back!"
   a) **Use**: Motivating the group toward improved relationships.
   b) **Underuse**: Ignoring other people's presence.
   c) **Overuse**: Welcoming superficially and ignoring tasks. Welcoming others while interrupting the group activity.

7. **LEVELERS**: "How do you feel about this? Be honest now!"
   a) **Use**: Promoting honest exchanges.
   b) **Underuse**: Withholding honest, relevant comments or requests for openness.
   c) **Overuse**: Pushing for openness prematurely or as avoidance of tasks.

8. **FOLLOWERS**: "I like what Susan just selected."
   a) **Use**: Listening and participating actively.
   b) **Underuse**: Failing to follow the group's procedures or being totally inactive.
   c) **Overuse**: Forcing conformity through the silent majority or apathetic following.

9. **OBSERVERS**: "I've noticed that we've always used voting as to decide things."
   a) **Use**: Noting and reporting on group progress.
   b) **Underuse**: Ignoring the group process.
   c) **Overuse**: Using observations to manipulate the group. Giving inaccurate or too detailed of a report.

Maintenance refers to group building and cohesiveness. It is very productive for each member to view maintenance as an important group goal, no matter what the group task. Sometimes groups overemphasize tasks and get very little done, due to the lack of good feelings needed, and the desire to spend the energy and time needed. Other groups underemphasize tasks, thus getting little accomplished while feeling very good about being together.

Individualistic Behaviors

Individualistic behaviors place member needs above group needs and interfere with task and maintenance. These behaviors may be caused by a low level of interpersonal skill, lack of interest, defensiveness, competition, ill-defined group goals and unproductive conflict.

Below is an example of each of the individualistic behaviors, together with the task and maintenance behaviors which could replace individualistic needs with productive behaviors, and the maintenance behaviors that would help the group and the individual cope with the strong individual needs.

Reducing Unhelpful Behaviors

1. **BLOCKERS**: "I don't think it will work. I won't support it."
   a) **Helpful task/maintenance replacement roles:**
Sharing reasons for blocking and the disadvantages which you see in the issue.
   b) **Helpful maintenance behaviors to cope with the individual needs:**
Leveling about feelings and asking group to help deal with them.

2. **AGGRESSORS**: "John, that is a dumb, dumb way to look at this!"

a) **Helpful maintenance replacement roles**

Expressing aggressive energy as encourager, standard setter, evaluator, or orienter.

b) **Helpful maintenance behaviors to cope with the individual needs:**

Describing aggressive feelings, leveling, setting standards, and working for cooperation.

3. **RECOGNITION SEEKERS**: "Here's a great idea I've used in the past."

a) **Helpful task/maintenance replacement roles:**

Getting attention to serve the necessary tasks, then giving attention to others through welcoming, encouraging, gate keeping, etc.

b) **Helpful maintenance behaviors to cope with the individual needs:**

Sharing feelings and facilitating the process regarding one's own needs and the needs of others.

4. **DOMINATORS**: "That'll never fly, Orville!"

a) **Helpful task/maintenance replacement roles:**

Energizing, evaluating, coordinating, standard setting, process facilitating, conflict managing.

b) **Helpful maintenance behaviors to cope with the individual needs:**

Leveling your own needs and feelings of certainty and uncertainty.

5. **AVOIDERS**: "I don't want to talk about this now. Can't we talk about it at the next meeting?"

a) **Helpful task/maintenance replacement roles:**

Relieving tension, orienting, coordinating, sharing opinions.

b) **Helpful maintenance behaviors to cope with the individual needs:**

Confronting group with the conflict stemming from the task and maintenance issues and one's resistance to change.

6. **SPECIAL INTEREST PLEADER**: "I think the group can do it this way, and it sure would help me in my work if we do."

a) **Helpful task/maintenance replacement roles:**

Leveling, encouraging, cooperating, facilitating the group process.

b) **Helpful maintenance behaviors to cope with the individual needs:**

Sharing one's own interests and how the group can help meet them and other's interests. This can be done during the group meeting and outside of the formal setting.

Each of us can try to be as positive a member as possible by replacing individualistic needs and behaviors with task and maintenance behaviors that are group-oriented. Sometimes one's own needs and feelings are very important and pull us toward individualistic action in one or more groups. When others in these groups can help us channel our behaviors into productive directions, it benefits all group members. In this way, groups can grow and try to help all members to meet important personal and "group" needs. Remember, we all have similar needs, so working together we "all" can benefit.

ACTIVITY 14–4

Select a team and observe the team's actions. In the space below, write a detailed description of the functional and dysfunctional behaviors you see, using the information on task, maintenance, and individualistic behaviors on pages 133 through 137 to assist you.

ACTIVITY 14–5

Examine the observation sheets on pages 140 to 141. They are set up to be useful in "tallying/counting" the number of task, maintenance, and individualistic contributions made by each team member, and most importantly by the entire team. Use one of the forms, or a copy of it, to observe a group meeting or work session. Write a short evaluation of the team's functioning and at least four recommendations that you would make for improvement.

Key points in evaluation:

1.

2.

3.

Recommendations for improvement:

1.

2.

3.

4.

OBSERVING TASK BEHAVIORS

Observer Name _____

Observation Date _____

Group Member Numbers

	1	2	3	4	5	6
Task Starting						
Initiators						
Information seekers						
Information givers						
Opinion seekers						
Opinion givers						
Procedural facilitators						
Doers						
Recorders						

	1	2	3	4	5	6
Task Accomplishment						
Orienters						
Elaborators						
Coordinators						
Evaluators						
Energizers						

OBSERVING MAINTENANCE BEHAVIORS

Observer Name _____

Observation Date _____

	Group Member Numbers					
	1	2	3	4	5	6
Maintenance						
Encouragers						
Gatekeepers						
Harmonizers						
Conflict Managers						
Standard Setters						
Welcomers						
Levelers						
Followers						
Observers						

OBSERVING INDIVIDUALISTIC BEHAVIORS

Observer Name _____

Observation Date _____

	1	2	3	4	5	6
Individualistic Behaviors						
Blockers						
Aggressors						
Recognition Seekers						
Dominators						
Avoiders						
Special Interest Pleaders						

ACTIVITY 14–6

Examine a work group that you are familiar with, either currently or from the past. Select two people you have worked with: one person with whom you enjoyed working, and one with whom you were very reluctant to work. For each person, list two behaviors that are characteristic of that person's interactions with others.

PERSON I USUALLY ENJOYED WORKING WITH	PERSON I WAS USUALLY RELUCTANT TO WORK WITH
1	1.
2.	2.

Next, respond to the following:

Do you demonstrate behaviors from either list?   YES   NO

Would you fall exclusively in one list or the other?   YES   NO

Cite two examples of your behavior to support your answer.

1.

2.

In considering the person you were reluctant to work with, cite two positive behaviors for him/her:

1.

2.

In what ways could you encourage growth and expansion of those behaviors?

1.

2.

What could this person contribute to a team?

1.

2.

ACTIVITY 14–7

Make a list of your strengths and weaknesses. Could any of your strengths ever interfere with a team process? Consider stereotypes such as the "rugged individualist" vs. the "teddy bear."

Strengths that could interfere with the team process:

1.

2.

Could any of your weaknesses ever expedite the team process? Why or why not? Cite examples:

1.

2.

ACTIVITY 14–8

Form a group of five students and complete the following exercises.

1. Make a list of several key team-building behaviors. Discuss the behaviors that produce high-performance teamwork on healthcare teams on which you and your classmates participate.

2. Working in teams with classmates who have similar group assignments or situations, develop an observation form with which you could evaluate the effectiveness of your teams outside of class. Set up a time to meet again once you have used the form and can talk about its usefulness and what you have observed about your teams.

People on a team have varied personalities and skills. An effective team draws on these individual skills to accomplish the task at hand. If all team members were clones, completing a task could prove difficult for each would be doing the same thing. The "Ivory Tower" activity that follows is designed to demonstrate that each person can contribute something unique to task accomplishment. For example, those strong in spatial relations may come up with a concept for the tower. Others whose strength lies in organization may demonstrate an ability to see that everyone is involved in helping to accomplish the task. Others may function as "cheerleaders" and energize the group. Be sure to note the different roles that everyone plays.

Team-Building Activity: THE IVORY TOWER

This activity can be done with one, two, or more groups of at least six persons. Two groups are preferred with others in an outer circle as silent observers, depending on the number of students in class.

Materials needed (each group):
1. colored construction paper (40–50 sheets)
2. masking tape
3. markers, either colored or black
4. two rolls of party streamers

Each group is to build a tower using the above materials only. They will have 30 minutes to construct the tower. They cannot discuss the construction until time begins. The group is solely responsible for delegating tasks, and deciding how the tower is to be built. The tower will be judged by the following criteria:
1. Height
2. Message; each tower must convey a message
3. Overall appearance

After the towers are built and "objectively" judged by a person who did not participate in the tower building, analyze the process by answering the following questions?
1. How did tasks get delegated? Did one person assume a leadership role? Did others willingly follow?
2. Was the goal clearly stated at the beginning? Did all the team members participate in deciding on the message as well as the structure? If not, was that okay with some of the members?
3. Did all team members participate in the process? How?
4. How did members differ in their participation? Were some more verbal than others? Were some more willing to participate in the actual construction? Was anyone "good" at all the tasks, assessing, planning, delegating, constructing? Did some team members focus on select tasks?
5. What was your part in the process? Were you comfortable with how the process worked? What suggestions would you have for yourself in similar situations in the future?
6. Did any team members assume a role that surprised you?

ACTIVITY 14–10

MINDMAPPING

Design a mindmap that represents the interlocking behaviors of members of an effectively functioning team. Identify how the behaviors of the entire team could be modified by one very individualistic or one very competitive member. What actions could the team take to maintain its integrity?

CHAPTER 15

EMPOWERING AND MOTIVATING STAFF

Joseph B. Hurst, Ph.D., Ed.D., and Mary J. Keenan, Ph.D., R.N.

INTRODUCTION

The word *empowerment* has different meanings for different people. It even made the 1992 list of trivial and meaningless terms, making it a part of the "gibberish" or jargon of today. How often have you heard people around you talking as though *empowerment* were a clear and easily understandable term? By examining the various meanings of this word, this chapter helps you determine how open, willing, and able you and others around you are to share power and to encourage others to take power and do something productive with it. The exercises in the first half of this chapter (Activities 15–1 through 15–8) help you determine how you tend to empower people now, and how you could continue to do so in the future.

The exercises in the second half of this chapter focus on risk taking as a key to coaching and empowerment. Two of the most important questions to ask yourself are, "How far can and should I go?" and "How big a risk can or should I take?" Activities 15–9 through 15–12 focus on your tendency to take risks and the factors that affect your risk taking.

OBJECTIVES

- To determine what actions would empower particular people in real and hypothetical situations.

- To assess your present patterns of empowerment and commit to an even more effective pattern for the future.

- To analyze situations that you find comfortable for taking risks and those in which you avoid risking.

- To practice giving and receiving positively framed feedback.

- To assess the degree to which you take risks and the personal and environmental factors that affect your risk taking.

- To analyze short case examples and determine how you might take appropriate risks and/or support others in doing so.

- To analyze the degree to which groups might be more or less supportive of risks and how a manager could promote appropriate levels of risk taking by others.

ACTIVITY 15–1

1. Write a short personal definition of the word empowerment.
   Empowerment means:

2. Review Chapter 15 in the textbook. Notice how empowerment is defined. Seek out two additional definitions of empowerment and identify how empowerment is defined.
   Reference:
   Empowerment is:

   Reference:
   Empowerment is:

3. Observe one to three people in your work or clinical setting. Identify at least three specific behaviors (examples) that demonstrate their willingness and ability to be responsible and accountable for completing action and producing results.
   Example:

   Example:

   Example:

   Cite two individual, supervisor, and/or team behaviors that promote and reinforce this willingness and ability to be responsible, accountable, and productive.
   Behavior:

   Behavior:

   Cite one way (example) that you can use to support empowerment for yourself and for another.
   Supportive example for self:

   Supportive example for another:

4. Cite specific statements of the behaviors you tend to display when you are intentionally and unintentionally empowering people. Start with yourself. What do you say, do, and/or think that empowers *you* when you need it?
   What I say:

   What I do:

   What I think:

What do you do and say that empowers *others* around you? (Include your supervisors, supervisees, peers, and patients.)

What I do:

What I say:

What I think:

5. Fill out the Present Empowerment Chart below, using your responses to the preceding questions as a guide. Consider your own and others' actions. What do you/they do, say, and think that empowers people around them? List specifically how you and others empower one another and allow yourselves to be empowered.

PRESENT EMPOWERMENT CHART

HOW DO I EMPOWER MYSELF?	HOW DO OTHERS EMPOWER ME?

HOW DO I EMPOWER OTHERS?	HOW DO OTHERS EMPOWER OTHERS?

ACTIVITY 15–2

1. Study the list of behaviors you developed in Activity 15–1 and any other resources you have regarding empowerment. Identify three new ways beyond those you identified in the Present Empowerment Chart with which you could empower people.

Ways to empower others in the clinical setting:

a)

b)

c)

2. Fill out the Future Empowerment Chart below, listing at least three new behaviors in each of the major sections. Transfer your answers from item 1 (above) of this activity to the appropriate section of the chart.

FUTURE EMPOWERMENT CHART

Consider your own and others' actions. What COULD you/they do, say, and think that WOULD empower people around them IN THE FUTURE? List specifically how you and others COULD empower one another and COULD allow yourselves to be empowered beyond what you do now.

HOW COULD I EMPOWER MYSELF?	HOW COULD OTHERS EMPOWER ME?
HOW COULD I EMPOWER OTHERS?	**HOW COULD OTHERS EMPOWER OTHERS?**

ACTIVITY 15–3

Meet in a group of three or four and fill out the Disempowerment Chart below. Focus on the specific beliefs, habits, regulations, and behaviors that tend to disempower nurses and nurse managers.

DISEMPOWERMENT CHART

Consider your own and others' actions. What do you/they do, say, and think that disempowers people around them? List specifically how you and others disempower one another and allow yourselves to be disempowered.

HOW DO I DISEMPOWER MYSELF?	HOW DO OTHERS DISEMPOWER ME?
HOW DO I DISEMPOWER OTHERS?	**HOW DO OTHERS DISEMPOWER OTHERS?**

ACTIVITY 15–4

In a group of three or four, discuss the behaviors you have written on the Present and Future Empowerment Charts (Activities 15–1 and 15–2) before class, comparing them with the behaviors you listed on the Disempowerment Chart (Activity 15–3). After your discussion, make two additional lists in the space below, choosing the three most important empowering behaviors that would *counteract* the disempowering behaviors, and the three most important behaviors that could *replace* them.

Counteracting behaviors:

1.

2.

3.

Replacement behaviors:

1.

2.

3.

ACTIVITY 15–5

Individually, commit yourself to a plan to behave in at least three new empowering ways. State specifically what behavior you will carry out, with whom, by when, and with what new results (e.g., "I will ask my supervisor what I could do to reduce her/his backlog of paperwork by the end of the week to reduce stress and delays").

1. I will

    with whom

    by when (date)

    with the new results

2. I will

    with whom

    by when (date)

    with the new results

3. I will

    with whom

    by when (date)

    with the new results

ACTIVITY 15–6

Examine and analyze typical dialogues among nurses, managers, and other health professionals. Cite three instances of both empowering and disempowering behaviors.

Empowering behaviors

1.

2.

3.

Disempowering behaviors

1.

2.

3.

Figure 15-1 below compares risk taking to a balance scale. The left side has space for you to list all the things about yourself personally that support or stimulate you to take risks at work. These factors might include such things as the degree to which you feel confident, able, dissatisfied, that you have nothing to lose, comfortable with change and challenge, stimulated to try something new, and a sense of self-esteem. Write statements moving from the lowest line up, as if you were adding weights to this side of the scale. Be specific and thorough in what you write so you are clearly describing what supports your risk taking (phrase it as you say it to yourself and/or others around you: e.g., "My attitude is that I can make it work."). List all the statements you can think of that positively affect your risk taking. Look at your list and star those three that "weigh" the most.

Next, on the right side of the figure, list the personal factors that block your risk taking at work. You could consider the degree to which you feel afraid, cautious, and unable to make mistakes; avoid looking foolish and/or try to be perfect; feel uncertain and uncomfortable; and try to please others. Again list specific statements from the bottom up, including those that most limit your risk taking. Then star the three that "weigh" the most.

7._____   7._____

6._____   6._____

5._____   5._____

4._____   4._____

3._____   3._____

2._____   2._____

1._____   1._____

Personal Factors That Support Risk Taking

Personal Factors That Block Risk Taking

Figure 15-1 Personal factors that support and block risk taking.

ACTIVITY 15–8

Figure 15–2 below is similar to Figure 15–1 from the preceding activity, but this time depicting environmental factors (external factors, or those that lie outside you) that affect your risk taking. In the spaces provided on the figure, write specific statements on the appropriate side of the diagram about the supportive or blocking effects of rules and laws, policies and procedures, others' opinions, economic issues, and safety issues. (For example, a supportive statement might be "My supervisor says to go for it," and a blocking statement might be "Public ridicule for past mistakes.")

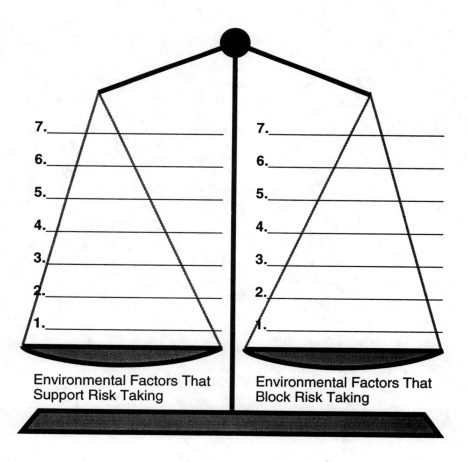

Figure 15-2 Environmental factors that support and block risk taking.

ACTIVITY 15–9

In the space below, write a short summary of how your personal balance scale tends to tip. When does it tip? Why? Identify whether you tend to be overly cautious, moderately cautious, careful in weighing the pros and cons, optimistic, or impulsive. Do you try to minimize your losses, or maximize your gains from any uncertain actions? Write a summary of what you discovered from looking at your scale and talking to other people about their risk taking, including just how risky it was for you to do these assignments.

ACTIVITY 15–10

Before class, discuss with three to five other students the balance scale diagrams you completed. Make a *group list* of the *top three* major personal and environmental blocking and supporting factors for taking risks to discover what all of you have learned about risk taking.

Supportive personal factors:

1.
2.
3.

Blocking personal factors:

1.
2.
3.

Supportive environmental factors:

1.
2.
3.

Blocking environmental factors:

1.
2.
3.

Use the following questions to guide your discussion:

1. What is risk taking and what affects the degree to which you tend to take risks?

2. How can you support others in taking appropriate risks? How can you get that same kind of support for yourself and others?

3. How and when does your risk taking have to change depending on the situations in which you find yourself as a manager? Why?

4. What new behaviors could you incorporate into your risk-taking style?

The purpose of this exercise is to experience the effects of providing positively framed feedback to your peers and to members of the nursing staff. The positively framed feedback that you share may be written on the form below for your reference. Focus your feedback on the recipients' leadership/membership behaviors.

1. Share both oral and written feedback with peers in your clinical learning group.
2. Choose one or more members of the nursing staff and share feedback with them.
3. Provide an example of positively framed feedback to *yourself* and share this with others in a clinical conference as they also share positively framed feedback about themselves.

On the Positively Framed Feedback Form below, list one positively framed behavior and one example of the behavior that you have identified (for sample statements, refer to the list of "Suggested Leadership/Membership Behaviors" that follows the form). In addition to the feedback you share with your peers, state at least one example for the staff nurse(s) that you have selected. Finally, state at least one positive behavior for yourself and one supporting example that you will share with your peers in the conference.

POSITIVELY FRAMED FEEDBACK FORM

For each person to whom you will be giving feedback, as well as yourself, state:

A.   One positive behavior that you would like to provide feedback about. Use behaviors from the list that follows or think of your own.

B.   One example or instance when you observed this person demonstrating the behavior you have identified.

1. Name:
   A. Behavior:
   B. Example:
2. Name:
   A. Behavior:
   B. Example:
3. Name:
   A. Behavior:
   B. Example:
4. Name:
   A. Behavior:
   B. Example:
5. Name:
   A. Behavior:
   B. Example:
6. Name:
   A. Behavior:
   B. Example:

7. Name:
   A. Behavior:
   B. Example:
8. Name:
   A. Behavior:
   B. Example:
9. Name:
   A. Behavior:
   B. Example:
10. Name (write your own name here):
    A. Behavior:
    B. Example:
11. Selected Staff Member:
    A. Behavior:
    B. Example:

SUGGESTED LEADERSHIP/MEMBERSHIP BEHAVIORS

I appreciate the way that you...

1.   stimulate quality and work with me to achieve it.
2.   show respect toward me and others.
3.   share your humor in tense situations.
4.   seek my ideas and use them when you can.
5.   offer help clinically.
6.   make me feel that my contributions are worthwhile.
7.   openly share your ideas.
8.   work collaboratively with others.
9.   seek suggestions from others and incorporate them.
10.   seek my suggestions and help me use them clinically.
11.   openly acknowledge accomplishments of others.
12.   consider my goals and ideas along with your own.
13.   incorporate feedback from others.
14.   give me specific, not general, feedback that I can use.
15.   stimulate my thinking and bring out the "best" in me.
16.   incorporate ideas of others and build on them.
17.   never "put me down" when offering critiques.
18.   actively seek clarification when in conflict situations.
19.   seek and use feedback from others.
20.   listen carefully to me and others (patients, nurses, etc.)
21.   openly share accurate information with others.
22.   provide support for others in group, clinically, etc.
23.   encourage and support others to meet goals.
24.   suggest ways for problem solving.
25.   share work responsibilities with others.

DISCUSSING POSITIVELY FRAMED FEEDBACK

Form a group either in or out of class and discuss the following:

1. What did it feel like when you were asked to formulate and offer positively framed feedback? Comfortable? Unusual? Normal? Uncommon?

2. How did it feel when the the other person responded to your feedback? Comfortable? Unusual? Normal? Uncommon?

3. How did you feel about sharing positively framed feedback to yourself in an open group? Comfortable? Unusual? Normal? Uncommon?

4. If you responded "comfortable" and "normal" or "unusual" and "uncommon," think about the norms of your group, about the norms of the work group? What are they? Do they support this type of feedback, is it offered frequently, or are they surprised by it? How many times did you hear people omit saying "Thank you" and instead say "That's my job" or "I do it all the time."

5. In your clinical/work setting, what kind of feedback do nurses tend to offer each other? You? Other students? How does the feedback given reflect the work group's norms? How does it support achievement of unit goals?

6. Can positively framed feedback also be used as a frame for "reprimands" or is it always complimentary?

7. Experiment with positive feedback as a frame for "reprimands."

8. Generate a list of "do's" and "dont's" in offering positively framed feedback. Give supporting examples.

MINDMAPPING

Construct a mindmap that depicts related behaviors, situations, and opportunities for empowering yourself and coaching others to accomplish solitary and mutual tasks and goals. Include specific behaviors that you can use in group situations to promote goal achievement.

CHAPTER 16

COMMUNICATING AND COLLABORATING

Joseph B. Hurst, Ph.D., Ed.D., Mary J. Keenan, Ph.D., R.N., Ann W. Baker, Ph.D., R.N., Marsha Brown, M.S.N., R.N., and Mary Ann Dimmick, M.S.N., R.N.

INTRODUCTION

Even the most devastating life experiences can be coped with effectively. Collaborative conflict resolution (see Chapter 17) and problem solving (see Chapter 6) are skills that are learned in ways similar to how other skills and behaviors are learned. Smart people recognize that they need help to better cope and they are motivated to change their usual methods of problem solving. The goal of Activities 16–1 through 16–3 is to explore the dynamics of identifying, supporting, and working toward a collaborative goal.

You have also been reading about the need for trust, the difficulties caused by distrust, and nurse manager's role in developing powerful relationships. Activities 16–4 through 16–7 are aimed at sharpening your abilities to acknowledge trusting relationships, diagnose difficulties with trust, and promote trust among the people around you.

OBJECTIVES

- **To develop and practice skills in collaboration.**

- **To identify, and act in, situations requiring collaboration.**

- **To examine the degree of trust in working relationships and determine how to increase trust where necessary.**

- **To commit to new behaviors that would promote trust in working relationships.**

ACTIVITY 16–1

Typical life experiences that nurses face daily may include:
1. feeling stuck in a job providing few opportunities for advancement
2. feeling humiliated after failing the CCRN certification examination
3. experiencing the responsibility of being an adult with aging parents
4. making a decision to terminate an unhappy marriage

Collegial support and assistance with problem solving is not only a professional responsibility, but also an effective way to contribute to the morale and productivity of the healthcare team.

You can complete this exercise in two ways. On your own, choose one of the examples above. (An example of number 1 might be a nurse who feels little satisfaction in a current position because it seems to have no opportunity for advancement.) List three personal reasons and/or behaviors that illustrate how your *discomfort (weaknesses)* and *comfort (strengths)* can influence your interaction with a colleague. Or, with a partner, choose and identify one typical life experience with a colleague that together you can analyze from the perspectives of both discomfort and comfort.

Uncomfortable	Comfortable
1. I don't want to be seen as interfering.	1. I feel that I'm empathic and a good listener.
2. Who am I to give advice? Advice leads to dependency and/or lack of accountability. What could I do to assist and support someone like her?	2. Jamie frequently talks to me about her work complaints and dissatisfaction. She even asked directly for my input and perspective on the issue.
3. She seems so much more intelligent than I am. Is she really interested?	3. I know that only Jamie can make a decision about what further actions she must take and by when.
4. I don't want her to feel angry or alienated.	4. I think I can be quite objective and supportive.
5. I don't know what words to use or how to start.	5. I can encourage her to be honest with me.
6. I don't really have any answers for her. I like my job and future outlook.	6. She needs to create some possibilities and alternatives for herself and I can assist her.

Use the same process for a problem you have recently encountered with a colleague. Make two lists similar to these above.

PROBLEM WITH A COLLEAGUE:

Uncomfortable	Comfortable

ACTIVITY 16–2

Problem definition: To determine "what is the problem," define the problem with a colleague that you selected in Activity 16-1 using the format below (review Activity 6-3 on workbook pages 50 and 51 for a discussion of this format).

1. Who and what is affected in what "problematic ways"?

2. Who and/or what is causing it?

3. What type of a problem is being confronted?
   As you see it:

   As others see it:

4. What are the intended goals/specific results to remedy the situation?

Meet with two to three classmates to discuss the "problem with a colleague" that you have identified. Now move forward to reflect, clarify your feelings, and further discuss and analyze the situation prior to identifying or initiating any subsequent action.

I'm uncomfortable about	I'm comfortable about
1.	1.
2.	2.
3.	3.
4.	4.
5.	5.

Personal or professional conflicts can be resolved in ways analogous to the nursing process. Suppose you are an expert in clinical problem solving. The first steps leading to collaboration are to identify the issue or problem (you've just done this, congratulations!) and then to identify strengths of the collaborator (you in this case).

ACTIVITY 16–3

ROLE PLAY
PARTICIPANTS

The participants are four role players, eight advisors/consultants (optional), and at least four observers, depending on the size of the group, as described below. (This role play could be repeated with groups of eight, using players and observers only depending upon the numbers of students in the class so that all could participate. It could also be done with only one group of participants and engaging the entire class as observers).

1. *Role Players.* Four volunteers to play the role parts. Role players are encouraged to embellish the roles and provide their own dialogue to heighten and "act out" the roles in keeping with the descriptions of the roles.

2. *Advisors/Consultants.* Four to eight additional volunteers (total, one or two for each role player) to provide advice or consultation prior to enacting the scenario. The two "consultant–advisors" are to be seated directly behind each of the role players, and may confidentially provide advice to the role players during the enactment.

3. *Observers.* Four to eight volunteers to assume the role of observers, take notes, and report back to the group about what was seen and heard. Observers should identify:

   a) goals of each role player
   b) areas of overlapping goals of role players
   c) overt and covert expressed feelings of role players
   d) what each participant wants from this meeting
   e) in what areas the participants were in agreement
   f) in what areas they disagreed

Part 1: Meeting 1—Setting the stage (Note: Each time this is enacted it will be different as the role players will modify it according to their own interpretations):

Role players: In a separate part of the classroom, each of the participants and their advisor–consultants should read and think about how to enact the roles. They should not share any part of the interpretation of the role with anyone following this confidential meeting.

Class: Review the components of collaboration. Discuss why collaboration is the most assertive and the most cooperative mode of conflict resolution. Review Chapter 16, and make a list of those behaviors you believe would be most helpful for a leader to approach a situation in a collaborative manner.

ROLES
Nurse Manager: Jeanne Smith

You are new on this unit. You were asked to work with this group to "bring them together." You are very effective in working with groups and you are very knowledgeable about using group skills, and combining this with your advanced knowledge about clinical nursing. You know that this group has a history of unresolved conflict, yet you know that each individual in the group is very knowledgeable and committed to the very highest standards. You also have recently learned that they have not been able to "pull it together," or to do very much other than to accomplish the minimum they need to do for the patients and their families. Most nurses in the unit are AD prepared and all are CCRN or ACLS certified. Your task is to bring them together to identify and carry out a unit-based quality-improvement project.

This is your first meeting with three members of the staff (selected by their peers). They know this meeting is to bring them together to request their assistance in identifying a group goal for a unit-based quality-improvement project.

Staff Nurses

Nancy Newsbetter: You have been working here for about 20 years. You have worked for several managers with several styles. They all try to "shake things up," yet nothing has changed much as far as you can see. It doesn't seem to matter what you say, they never listen anyway. Managers come and go. Now they want you to do something else. "This, too, shall pass." You would really like to be heard, and have others incorporate your ideas into the unit goals.

Jo Ellen Jones: You have been on this unit for about two years. You seem to be the only one who cares. Furthermore, you are the only one who really works around here. You would like to have others "do their share." The others are good, but... They just don't seem to be interested in your ideas, only their own. That means that you have to do everything yourself, if you want it done. You would really like to be heard, and to work with someone else.

John Done: You are new on this unit. You were on one similar to this when you were in the Army. The nurses here are very competent, yet they don't seem happy with their accomplishments. You are still finding your way around. Although everyone seems to want to work with you, they all seem to want to do it on their own terms. They don't seem to want to listen to you. You would really like to be heard and to participate in identifying and meeting the unit goals. They just don't seem to be very well organized.

Part 2: Meeting 2—Setting the Stage:

Jeanne Smith, the nurse manager, returned to her office on the nursing unit to determine what to do next. She reviewed the proceedings of the previous meeting as well as the feedback from the observers. She determined that one area in which all participants were in agreement was that nobody "listened" to them. She also noted that frequently the staff nurses openly and covertly implied that they did not feel that their input was valued. She used these ideas and called the second meeting to discuss the feedback and to determine "where do we go from here?" She also sat back and looked at whom we thought were the "stakeholders" in this project. At this point we decided to look at this aspect and move toward redefining a broad, common, superordinate goal. Having outlined new goals for the next meeting, she then proceeded to outline a process whereby they could all move forward.

After the meeting, the staff nurses gathered around and discussed their meeting with their new manager. They discussed how it had always been, wondering how it could change. Then they moved on to discuss how they would like it to be, and how they could function differently. They heard from the nurses on other units that the entire nursing department would be doing unit-based quality-improvement projects and questioned if this was another "fly-by-night" project, and if it was something that they would all be required to participate in? They also wondered if the new nurse manager was trustworthy. Did she really mean what she said, or is this just like all the rest of the "busy work" dreamed up by somebody else who didn't really care about what they thought. They decided tentatively that maybe it was worth a try, but they wanted to hear more before they committed to this or any other project.

DEBRIEFING

1. Cite three turning points in this discussion.
   a)
   b)
   c)
2. Cite two actions of the nurse manager toward establishing a superordinate (collaborative) goal.
   a)
   b)
3. State two concerns of the staff nurses.
   a)
   b)
4. How might this have been handled differently?

   Why?
   What other outcomes could have resulted?
   a) Positive

   b) Negative

5. Who were two of the stakeholders in this scenario?
   a)
   b)
   Why?
   What "stakes" were they holding?

   What did they want to preserve?

   What were they willing to give up?

   Why?
6. Cite at least two reasons that you think they modified their previous position and decided to become more cooperative.
   a)

   b)

7. In what areas (ways) were the staff and the manager cooperative? Assertive?
   Staff Cooperation:
   a)
   b)
   Staff Assertiveness:
   a)
   b)
   Manager Cooperation:
   a)
   b)
   Manager Assertiveness:
   a)
   b)

ANALYZING AND DEVELOPING TRUSTING RELATIONSHIPS

Read the "Characteristics of the Four C's" included in this activity. In the spaces below, list at least three characteristics of the behavior of people you tend to trust.

People whom I trust generally are/do:

1.
2.
3.

Think about your own characteristics and behavior from the perspectives of people with whom you work.

People at work whom I trust generally are/do:

1.
2.
3.

CHARACTERISTICS OF THE "FOUR C' S"

COMMON GROUND

The common ground in a trust relationship may be narrow, such as trusting the television repair person to fix the television. In many cases, such as friendships, marriages, and key working relationships, the common ground can be very broad and essential to well-being. It is very important to know the common ground in a trust relationship.

For instance, in working relationships, common ground can be the "reason for being" or a mission statement of the organization, task interdependence and common objectives, a shared history, etc...

COMPETENCE

The areas of competence necessary for trust can vary widely depending on the specific nature of the relationship. It is important, however, for those areas to be identified and affirmed. It helps both parties in the trust relationship.

CHARACTER

There are a variety of elements (or "characteristics") that can play a role in the perception of character. Some of them include honesty, perseverance, will, humor, clear beliefs and values, action orientation, accepting, caring, vision, etc... There are, obviously, many more "characteristics" that can impact trust. The more clear the partners in a trust relationship are about the "characteristics" that are important to them, the more control they can have over the degree of trust they can create.

CONSISTENCY

Competence and character that are demonstrated consistently supports the "leap of faith" necessary for trust. Trust can be lost very quickly through erratic or contradictory behavior and through a lack of consistent confidentiality. People need to know that their private matters are respected and held in strict confidence.

In the spaces below list at least four of your characteristics and behaviors that would promote trust and two that could promote distrust from others around you.

Trust-promoting behaviors:

1.

2.

3.

4.

Trust-inhibiting behaviors:

1.

2.

ACTIVITY 16–5

Read the directions for drawing a trust network on page 174 of this workbook. Use colored pencils or pens to draw a network of the important relationships you have in your clinical or work setting. Place the circles with people's initials in the appropriate third (superiors, peers, subordinates; see page 175) at a distance from "self" in the middle that visually represents the "distance" or "closeness" of that relationship. As the instructions suggest, draw lines that represent the importance of the relationship; indicate the degree of trust you each have toward one another; somewhere near the relationship lines you have drawn, write terms that describe the nature of the relationship. Analyze your network diagram and write several conclusions you can draw from the pattern(s) you observe. Think realistically about these relationships and their strengths and weaknesses.

Conclusions:

Complete the Trust Planning Worksheet on page 176 of this workbook. List three important people (could be a team) selected from your "network of professional relationships" in column 1. (Leave several blank lines between their names or initials.) In column 2 list major elements of your relationship with that person or team that are "working" (going well) and some that are "missing" (could be added). In column 3 list behaviors you could expand or add to how you act in the relationship that would increase trust and effectiveness.

Now, using the space below, create an action plan in which you commit to actions you have identified; take the actions, and observe what happens. Notice your own and others' barriers to trusting.

INSTRUCTIONS FOR DRAWING A TRUST NETWORK

A trust network is simply a visual representation of your trust relationships. Those relationships can be with superiors, peers, or subordinates. Such a picture can give you a great deal of insight very quickly into their importance and degree of trust.

ELEMENTS OF A NETWORK:

1. *The people*-Identify the people with whom you have key working relationships by initials and name in a circle.
2. *Relationship lines*-Draw lines from self to each person and from each person to self. Indicate by type of line (width, broken, squiggle, etc...), by distance, and by color and numbers (1) the importance of the relationship (your assessment and how you think the other person would assess it) and (2) the level of trust (your assessment and how you think the other would assess it).
3. *Descriptive words*-Key trust practices or building blocks can be added or adjectives and adverbs can be used to characterize the key relationship. List them near the lines representing each particular relationship.
4. Create a "key" at the bottom to remind yourself of what everything means.

Things about trust to remember or explore further:

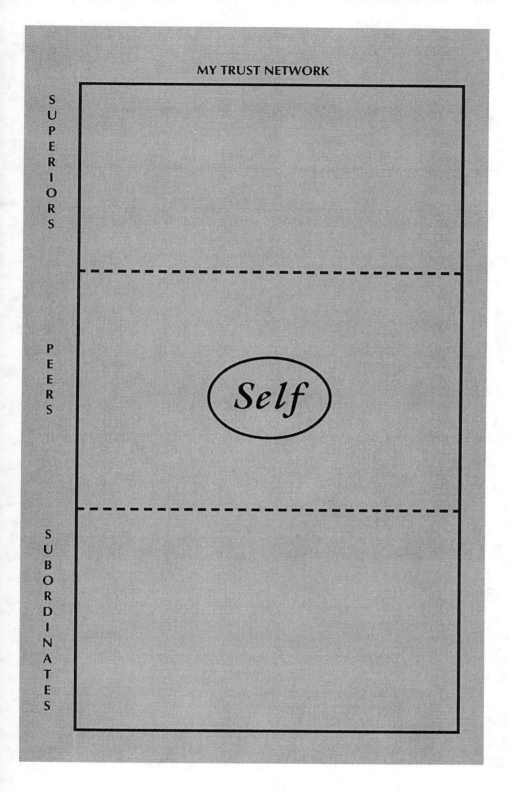

TRUST PLANNING WORKSHEET

With whom are your most important trust relationships?	What is currently working and what is currently missing in those relationships?	What actions/practices would be necessary to strengthen those trust relationships?

ACTIVITY 16–6

Meet in groups of two or three. Discuss your trust network diagrams and Trust Planning Worksheets.

What affects or influences my ability to trust the most?

1.

2.

Why?

List two ways I can increase trust in myself and in my colleagues.

1.

2.

List two ways to support one another in committing to and taking the actions listed in column 3 of the worksheet.

1.

2.

ACTIVITY 16–7

In the space below or on a large sheet of paper, create a collage, chart, or drawing that depicts the major trust factors you have identified. Present this to the rest of the class or small group and listen to what others have identified.

ACTIVITY 16–8

1. Meet in pairs. Discuss the characteristics and behaviors you tend to trust and distrust.

2. Take a scarf, handkerchief, or blindfold and put it over the eyes of one partner. Flip a coin or draw straws to decide who goes first. Take a walk for 10 minutes in which the sighted partner leads the other around, down the hall, out of the room, etc. Notice how you feel, what things you say to one another, and the considerations you have about other people. Discuss trust as you go. After you have walked for 10 minutes, change the blindfold to the other partner and return to the classroom taking a new route, and observe your feelings, thoughts, concerns, and trust. CAUTION: CONSIDER AND OBSERVE SAFETY PRECAUTIONS THROUGHOUT THIS ACTIVITY WHILE YOU EXPERIMENT WITH TRUSTING ONE ANOTHER.

3. Discuss with a small group:

a) What did I personally discover about my own tendencies to trust and be trustworthy?

b) What did we as a pair discover about our tendencies to trust each other as we progressed through this activity? Why did this happen?

c) What have we all discovered about trust that will be useful in our communication and collaboration in nursing, teaming, and managing?

MINDMAPPING

Devise a way of portraying graphically the various behaviors that contribute to and are integral portions of collaborative goal setting and collaborative goal achievement. Include components from previous chapters, such as communication, coaching, motivating, and empowerment so that the map depicts interrelationships among the supportive behaviors that you have identified. Include actions that nurses (individually and collectively) can take to promote collaboration.

CHAPTER 17

MANAGING CONFLICT

Joseph B. Hurst Ph.D., Ed.D., and Mary J. Keenan,
Ph.D., R.N.

INTRODUCTION

Conflict is a common and potentially productive aspect of working together in teams, one–to–one relationships, and organizations. The purpose of this chapter is to focus on ways to analyze conflicts and their progress and then to take action to match the most appropriate approach to the conflict.

OBJECTIVES

*   **To determine the nature of actual and hypothetical conflicts and decide how to resolve them.**

*   **To develop skills in assisting others to resolve conflicts in which they are engaged.**

*   **To expand insight into personal behavior and determine preferred ways of resolving conflict.**

ACTIVITY 17–1

After you have read Chapter 17 in the textbook, complete and score the Conflict Self-Assessment on pages 344–346 in the text. Next, write out your responses to the self–assessment questions for each of the five approaches to conflict on pages 347, 348, 349, 350, and 352 of the textbook (avoiding, accommodating, competing, compromising, and collaborating), focusing only on conflicts in your professional life. (If you are not yet in a professional position, you might instead focus on conflicts during your "career" as a student.) Use the Conflict Reflection Form below to focus your thinking. What new behaviors have you committed to for the future?

CONFLICT REFLECTION FORM

Look at your scores on the Conflict Self-Assessment and responses to the five sets of self–assessment questions in the textbook. Reflect on how you act during conflict (professional and/or personal). Be honest with yourself without being critical.

1. How do you tend to balance the following polarities related to conflict?
    a) Unassertiveness and assertiveness?
    b) Uncooperativeness and cooperativeness?
    c) Avoidance and involvement?
    d) Escalating and minimizing any conflict?
    e) Rigid control and loose improvisation?
    f) Revealing and concealing information?
    g) Intellectual and emotional reactions?

2. Which two approaches to conflict resolution do you tend to underemphasize? Why?
    a)

    b)

3. Which two do you tend to use most frequently? Why?
    a)

    b)

4. How might you be overemphasizing some approaches? Are they situation specific, or are they just the ones you rely on? Why?

5. When and how might you be matching approaches effectively to the particular nature of conflicts in which you are involved?

6. When and how might you be matching approaches ineffectively with the particular nature of conflicts in which you are involved?

ACTIVITY 17–2

Another copy of the Conflict Assessment from your textbook appears below. Complete it again, this time focusing on your personal life. While responding to each statement in the assessment, think of how you act in personal conflicts with your family and friends. Score and reflect on your personal pattern of approaches to conflict. What strengths, weaknesses, and missing actions do you notice? How are your personal and professional patterns similar and different?

CONFLICT ASSESSMENT

Directions: Read each of the statements below. Assess yourself in terms of how frequently you tend to act that way during conflict at work. Place the number of the most appropriate response in the blank in front of each statement: 1 if the behavior is never typical of how you act during a conflict; 2 if it is seldom typical; 3 if it is occasionally typical; 4 if it is frequently typical; or 5 if it is very typical of how you act during conflict. Please complete all items.

_____ 1. Create new possibilities to address all important concerns.
_____ 2. Persuade others to see it and/or do it my way.
_____ 3. Work out some sort of give-and-take agreement.
_____ 4. Let other people have their way.
_____ 5. Wait and let the conflict take care of itself.
_____ 6. Find ways that everyone can win.
_____ 7. Use whatever power I have to get what I want.
_____ 8. Find an agreeable compromise among people involved.
_____ 9. Give in so others will get what they think is important.
_____ 10. Withdraw from the situation.
_____ 11. Assertively cooperate until everyone's needs are met.
_____ 12. Compete until I either win or lose.
_____ 13. Engage in "give a little and get a little" bargaining.
_____ 14. Make others needs met over my own needs.
_____ 15. Avoid taking any action for as long as I can.
_____ 16. Partner with others to find the most inclusive solution.
_____ 17. Put my foot down assertively for a quick solution.
_____ 18. Negotiate for what all sides value and can live without.
_____ 19. Agree with what others want to create harmony.
_____ 20. Keep as far away from others involved as possible.
_____ 21. Stick with it to get everyone's highest priorities.
_____ 22. Argue and debate over the best way.
_____ 23. Create some middle position everyone agrees to.
_____ 24. Put my priorities below those of the other people.
_____ 25. Hope the issue does not come up.
_____ 26. Collaborate with others to achieve our goals together.
_____ 27. Compete with others for scarce resources.
_____ 28. Emphasize compromise and trade-offs.
_____ 29. Cool things down by letting others do it their way.
_____ 30. Change the subject to avoid the fighting.

CONFLICT ASSESSMENT SCORING

Look at the numbers you placed in the blanks on the conflict assessment on the previous page. Write the number you placed in each blank on the appropriate line below. Add up your total for each column, and enter that total on the appropriate line. The greater your total for each approach, the more frequently you tend to use that approach to conflict at work. The lower the score, the less frequently you tend to use that approach to conflict at work.

Collaborating	Competing	Compromising	Accommodating	Avoiding
1._____	2._____	3._____	4. _____	5._____
6._____	7._____	8._____	9. _____	10. _____
11. _____	12. _____	13. _____	14. _____	15. _____
16. _____	17. _____	18. _____	19. _____	20. _____
21. _____	22. _____	23. _____	24. _____	25. _____
26. _____	27. _____	28. _____	29. _____	30. _____
Total ____	Total ____	Total ____	Total _____	Total ____

Throughout the rest of this section, there are descriptions of each approach and related self-assessment and commitment-to-action activities. Use these totals to stimulate your thinking about how you do and could handle conflict at work. Most importantly, consider if your pattern of frequency tends to be consistent, or inconsistent, with the types of conflicts you face. That is, does your way of dealing with conflict tend to match the situations in which that approach is most useful.

ACTIVITY 17–3

In the space below, write a creative short story that describes your approach to professional conflicts. Be imaginative and let yourself go, while summarizing for yourself and others what you see regarding your reactions to conflict. Suspend any negative self–judgment you have about being creative or using your intuitive side. Emphasize actions and outcomes.

PLAYING TWENTY QUESTIONS: CONFLICT ANALYSIS

Reflect on past and present conflicts in which you have been directly involved. Choose one conflict to focus on, particularly if it seems to be reappearing with the same or with other people. Check the textbook to determine whether it is a polarity. If it is, choose another conflict that is not a polarity. Then, write out your responses to each of the twenty questions below.

DEFINING THE CONFLICT

1. Who was the conflict between? How were they affected?
   Who:
   How:
   Who:
   How:
2. Who else was affected and how?
   Who:
   How:
3. What was the actual conflict? What were the perceived incompatibilities?

CONFLICT PROCESS ANALYSIS

Frustration Stage

4. What did you feel at the start and in the early stages of the conflict?

5. Why did you feel this way?

6. How did you act as a result of these feelings?

7. What did the other people feel at the start and in the early stages of the conflict?

8. Why did they feel this way?

9. How did they act as a result of these emotions?

10. After the conflict moved into the conceptualization stage (see below), what other emotions, or changes in your initial emotions, occurred? Why?

Conceptualization Stage

11. What did you think the real conflict or issue, fight, disagreement, etc., was? Why?

12. What do you think now that the other people believed the conflict, or issue, fight, disagreement, etc., was? Why?

13. Where did you and others have serious differences: facts and information, goals and objectives, means and methods of action, and/or standards and values?

14. Describe why you had the following differences:
    a) Exposure to different data

    b) Different interpretations of the information

    c) Differences in your roles and position

    d) Different values and beliefs

    e) Cultural differences

    f) Different orders from someone else?

15. After the conflict moved into the action stage, what new views of the conflict (conceptualizations) were created by anyone involved? Why?

Action

16. How did you act specifically (and which of the five approaches to conflict were tried)? Why?

17. How did the other people act? Why?

18. After the conflict clearly was in the outcome stage, were there any new actions by anyone that were aimed as resolving this conflict or in changing any of the outcomes below?

Outcomes

19. What happened to the quality of task accomplishment and efficiency of action as a result of the actions taken? Why?

20. What happened to the quality of the relationships among those involved?

ACTIVITY 17–5

Imagine that you will be in a conflict in the future similar to the one you just analyzed in Activity 17–4. Knowing what you do about this past conflict, your tendencies to approach conflict (review the self–assessments in Chapter 17 of the textbook), and the five different approaches to conflict, write out a short scenario below (including all four stages of the process) describing how you could act to resolve the conflict.

ACTIVITY 17–6

1. Select a partner and meet to discuss what you have discovered about yourself regarding conflict in Activities 17–1 through 17–5. Focus on and cite three of your strengths, new possibilities, and commitments to new action.

   a)

   b)

   c)

   Review the five approaches to conflict resolution and create a short realistic case-study scenario based upon the use of one of them. As a pair, reflect upon your clinical experiences and select an example from a recent one. Be specific so that you can meet with another pair to share and gain their insight to decide upon an approach for resolution. Briefly identify:

   Who? You and

   What was the conflict as you saw it?

   What was the conflict as the other person saw it?

   When did the conflict occur?

   Where did the conflict occur?

   Why do you think the conflict occurred?

   Why did the other person think the conflict occurred?

2. Choose a pair of students to meet with you and your partner. Serve as the other pair's conflict case/scenario editors, and then have them do the same for you. Read each other's cases, considering their clarity, realism, completeness, open-endedness, and appropriateness in terms of conditions and conflict approach. Assist each other in improving your cases.

3. Find another group of four, and exchange your group's two cases with their two cases. In your original pairs, take one of the two cases, read it, and decide what the real conflict is and how it could best be resolved. Then, meet again in your group of four and discuss your suggestions for both cases, making any necessary additions. Finally, get the suggested approaches from the original authors of your case and compare and contrast your responses.

4. Identify and discuss at least five specific questions and discoveries that your group has made resulting from this exercise.

   a)

   b)

   c)

   d)

   e)

DEBATE

Find a partner. One of you will assume the role (position) of a nurse manager, and the other, the role (position) of "devil's advocate" (i.e., taking the opposing view). Debate the issues described below, identifying the facts and fallacies of the debate and utilizing the chapter references to support or refute your conclusions. Do you agree or disagree with the following statements?

1. Conflict includes the talked-about problem and the other (real problem).

2. Most (or few) employees want managers to solve their problems for them.

3. The real difficulty with conflict lies in the way people experience the problem.

4. Nursing managers may sometimes be intensely uncomfortable about counseling/setting limits with employees.

ACTIVITY 17–8

Before class, create and write out or find some realistic case studies that need conflict resolution. Find at least one pertinent and relatively difficult case. Before starting this activity, quickly review what you have learned about conflict, the five approaches, and the potential outcomes. Bring your case studies to class and complete the following steps:

1. Set up two labeled boxes (envelopes, etc.), one to hold the difficult cases and the other to hold the other cases. Either individually, in a pair, or in a small group, draw a case (difficult or other) and prepare to either discuss it or role play how the case could be best resolved. (If you do this exercise in a group, you might want to rehearse it before class.) Carry out your discussion or role play either in front of the entire class or before smaller groups within the class, such as clinical conference groups in which more than one case is presented at a time.

2. Present your case resolutions and conduct a debriefing discussion after each case.

3. Summarize important principles and possibilities.

MINDMAPPING

Think about a very recent conflict that you have experienced. Draw a mindmap that illustrates the components that you recall, e.g., frustration. Compare your mindmap with the components of conflict identified in the textbook chapter. To this add the additional dimensions discussed in the chapter that you may have omitted as well as the modes of resolution. Make some suggestions and resolutions for handling confict the next time you encounter it.

CHAPTER 18
MANAGING PERFORMANCE

Neil VanderVeen, Ph.D.

INTRODUCTION

This chapter discusses the importance of performance appraisal and the advantages and disadvantages of various measurement instruments that can be used to evaluate performance. Just as important as the instrument is the emotional and physical environment in which the appraisal meeting takes place. This chapter provides you with an opportunity to practice some of the skills necessary for effective performance appraisal.

OBJECTIVES

*   **To understand differences among instruments that are used for performance appraisal.**

*   **To increase awareness of the importance of the emotional environment in performance appraisal.**

*   **To enable objective evaluation of performance appraisal processes.**

ACTIVITY 18–1

Design a performance appraisal process that you believe would help you to grow professionally.

1. Which of the performance appraisal types listed below would be a part of your preferred process? In the spaces below, identify the strengths and limitations of each. State a rationale for each regarding how the process could help you professionally.
   a) *Graphic rating scales* provide feedback that can:

   Strengths:
   Limitations:
   b) *Forced distribution* provides feedback that can:

   Strengths:
   Limitations:
   c) *Peer review* provides feedback that can:

   Strengths:
   Limitations:
   d) *Management by objectives* provides feedback that can:

   Strengths:
   Limitations:
   e) *Behaviorally Anchored Rating Scales* provide feedback that can:

   Strengths:
   Limitations:

2. State three performance criteria that should be included in your process.
   a)
   b)
   c)

3. Meet with one to three students to construct a performance appraisal form incorporating each of the performance criteria that you have identified.

4. Share the group process that has been developed with a person responsible for appraising you, or someone who would. Will that person agree to use your process to assist you to grow professionally? Remember, because your organization uses a particular system, that does not preclude the use of an *additional* system!

Assess the state of performance appraisal in a clinical organization (setting) by using the checklist below.

____ 1. Does your organization have a formal performance appraisal system? (If "no", see last item on this list.)
____ 2. Does it use graphic rating scales?
____ 3. Does it use forced distribution?
____ 4. Does it include peer review?
____ 5. Is it based on management by objectives?
____ 6. Are the objectives based on a strategic plan?
____ 7. Does it include a behaviorally anchored rating scale?
____ 8. Does it influence compensation?
____ 9. Does it serve as the basis for discipline?
____ 10. It is used to determine training needs?
____ 11. Does it increase role clarity?
____ 12. Do appraisal meetings occur at least quarterly?
____ 13. Is the system based on up-to-date position descriptions/criteria?
____ 14. Is there a clearly defined training process for appraisers?
____ 15. Every organization has an appraisal process! If your organization has no formal process, you can be sure that an informal process exists. Your performance is assessed!

Cite three examples of criteria used in the informal system in the organization.
1.
2.
3.

What is your opinion regarding the workings of the informal system of appraisal in your organization?

How does the informal system of performance appraisal reflect the values, climate, or cultural of the setting? Cite two ways.
1.
2.

ACTIVITY 18–2

This activity consists of developing a process for appraising the performance of your class instructor. Remember, a fair appraisal instrument looks forward, not backward. It would be unfair to judge your instructor's performance on criteria that were developed after the fact.

1. Meet in groups with four to six members. Develop a list of behaviors that are required of the instructor. For example, you may believe that faculty should provide a clear description of course grading criteria. List the proposed performance criteria for faculty teaching behaviors generated by your group.

   a)

   b)

   c)

   d)

   e)

2. Present your list of behaviors to another group. Behavioral statements state what the person must do to demonstrate accomplishment. They are not value laden. Stating what must be done to evidence that an assignment/achievement has been accomplished would generate behaviorally anchored criteria. Example: A score of 90 percent or higher will result in an "A" for the course is a behavioral statement. Stating that an "A" can be achieved with "quality" writing is not behavioral as the components are not clearly identified for what is meant by "quality." If criteria statements are not behavioral and objective then measurement will be a problem for it is dependent upon individual interpretation.

3. Request your course faculty (the university employee in this case) to respond to each of the behaviors that your group has generated in terms of fairness, objectivity, and appropriateness to the role of university faculty responsibility in this course.

ACTIVITY 18–3

1. Now that you have identified behavioral criteria for faculty in this course, it is only fair and appropriate to establish behaviorally anchored criteria for your student performance in this course. Meet in groups of four to six students. Each group is to develop a list of five behaviors that are required of the students, for example, completing assigned readings on time. List the student behaviors generated by your group.

   a)

   b)

   c)

   d)

   e)

2. Present your group's list of behaviors to the total group and to the faculty for feedback. Statements that are not behavioral should be clearly identified because if they are not behavioral, objectivity and measurement will be a problem. The faculty will provide feedback on how complete the lists are and on how measurable the items are.

ACTIVITY 18–4

1. Form a group of six to eight to brainstorm a list of behaviors that will produce a positive emotional environment (good feeling, productive) and behaviors that will produce a negative environment (bad feeling, punitive) during an appraisal session. Include both verbal and nonverbal behaviors (cues) that can contribute to creating supportive and nonsupportive environments. List the positive and negative behaviors generated by your list below.

Positive Behaviors   **Negative Behaviors**

2. Ask for two volunteers from each group, one to play the role of appraiser and one to play the role of appraised. Use the descriptors generated above for both positive and negative environments. The situational context will be the following classroom behaviors:
   a) arriving at class on time
   b) actively participating in classroom discussion
   c) supporting the ideas of other students in the class
   d) appropriately challenging the opinions (not facts) presented by the instructor

3. In conducting the *first* appraisal session, have the appraiser use only behaviors from the negative list above and none of the behaviors from the positive list. Observe and record five verbal and nonverbal reactions of the person being appraised:
   a)
   b)
   c)
   d)
   e)
   At the end of the appraisal session have the observers share their observations with the group.

4. Repeat the appraisal session, but this time have the appraiser use only behaviors from the positive list and none of the behaviors from the negative list. Again, note and record five verbal and nonverbal reactions of the person being appraised:
   a)
   b)
   c)
   d)
   e)
   At the end of the appraisal session, again have observers share their observations with the group.

ACTIVITY 18–5

MINDMAPPING

Envision yourself as the person responsible for developing a new performance appraisal procedure that will be uplifting emotionally and a way of increasing productive output for all—managers and employees. Draw a mindmap depicting current systems of performance apraisal, including the foci, purposes, outputs, and emotional highs and lows for each system. Look at managerial and employee comforts and discomforts with each type of appraisal. Now form a group, share your ideas, and collectively create the ideal performance appraisal system.

CHAPTER 19

MANAGING PERSONAL/ PERSONNEL PROBLEMS

Rosalind M. Peters, M.S.N., R.N.

INTRODUCTION

Successfully managing personal/personnel problems is a crucial element of the role of a nurse manager. To master this role function requires that the manager be able to accurately identify personnel problems, develop intervention strategies, implement those strategies, and then evaluate the effectiveness of the interventions. The exercises in this chapter will help you develop the assessment and intervention skills necessary to successfully manage personnel problems.

OBJECTIVES

- **To examine common personal and personnel problems.**

- **To determine agency policies and procedures related to substance abuse employees.**

- **To describe the factors involved in substance dependence and abuse problems.**

- **To determine professional nursing standards regarding substance abuse nurses.**

- **To examine legal, ethical, and personal issues related to terminating an employee.**

- **To determine the impact of role stress in the workplace.**

PERSONAL/PERSONNEL PROBLEMS: CHEMICAL DEPENDENCY

1. Review the following documents:

   a) Your state board of nursing's policy and procedure regarding chemically impaired nurses.

   b) The American Nurses' Association *Code for Nurses* and the policy statement regarding chemical dependency.

   c) A healthcare agency's policy and procedures regarding chemically dependent employees.

   d) A healthcare agency's policy regarding employees drug screening.

2. Define the differences between substance dependence and substance abuse.

Substance dependence is:

Substance abuse is:

3. List three factors leading to substance abuse in employees.

   a)

   b)

   c)

4. List five of the most common types of abused substances.

   a)

   b)

   c)

   d)

   e)

5. Describe four signs and symptoms of dependence/abuse that may be evident in a chemically impaired employee.

   a)

   b)

   c)

   d)

6. Write a short paragraph either supporting or contesting the following statements regarding chemically impaired healthcare employees.

   a) Substance dependence/abuse is a disease and therefore not fully under the control of the affected person. Substance abusers should be treated, not punished.

b) Nurses and other health professionals with their knowledge about drugs as well as their social contract with patients should be held to higher standards than the general population.

7. Obtain a copy of personnel policies from an agency in which you have clinical experience. Analyze the policy in relation to the following factors, recording your answers in the space provided.
a) Is the *Diagnostic and Statistical Manual* (*DSM-IV*) definition used to define substance dependence/abuse in the agency policy?

b) Is there a policy for reporting suspected or known impaired employees? If so what is the role of the nurse manager? Staff nurse?

c) Does the policy include plans for intervention and treatment? Is an employee assistance program (EAP) provided for employees? What is the manager's role in intervention?

d) Does the policy include notification procedure? If so, who within the agency administration is to be notified? What is the policy for notifying the state board of nursing if the impaired worker is a nurse?

e) List three key elements that you think should be included in an "ideal" agency policy.

PERSONAL/PERSONNEL PROBLEMS: MANDATORY DRUG TESTING FOR HEALTHCARE PROFESSIONALS

1. Review a copy of the following documents:

   An agency's policy and procedure regarding chemically dependent employees.

   An agency's policy regarding employee preemployment and on-the-job drug screening.

   Your state board of nursing's policy and procedure on reporting suspected chemically dependent nurses.

   The American Nurses' Association *Code for Nurses*. Determine their policy statement regarding substance abuse.

   An agency's policies on nondiscrimination in employment under the Americans with Disabilities Act.

2. Prepare to debate the issue of mandatory drug testing for healthcare employees. Read the following debating statement. Prepare five key points to argue for each side (pro and con) of the issue, drawing support for your arguments from the list of readings in item 1 above. Whereas approximately 70 percent of all cases handled by state boards of nursing are related to chemically impaired nurses, and Whereas nurses have entered into a social contract with their clients to provide safe care, Therefore, mandatory, random drug testing should be done on all practicing nurses.

PRO	CON
a)	
b)	
c)	
d)	
e)	

ACTIVITY 19-3

1. Read about the legal, regulatory, and ethical issues related to termination of an employee. Refer to the following readings as a guide.

> Faltermeyer, E. (1992). Is this layoff necessary? *Fortune.* 125(11): 71-72, 86.
>
> Wise, L. (1993). The erosion of nursing resources: Employee withdrawal behaviors. *Research in Nursing and Health Care.* 16(1):67-65.
>
> Brockner, J., Grover, S., Reed, T., and DaWitt, R. (1992). Layoffs, job-insecurity, and survivors work effort: Evidence of an inverte-U relationship. *Academy of Management Journal.* 35(-2): 413-425.

2. Review an agency's policies and procedures for terminating employees.
3. Read the scenario below. Carefully weigh the pros and cons of each termination decision, considering the legal, ethical, and personal factors that enter into your decision.

DOWNSIZING SCENARIO

You are a nurse manager in an agency that is experiencing financial difficulties. This problem affects more than just your agency. You are located in a county that is economically depressed and unemployment is high. You have just received the budget for the next financial year and note that you have lost one full-time position, meaning you must lay off one of your full-time nurses. Due to the poor economic situation, it is not possible to transfer within the agency and the layoff will most likely be a permanent one. Also, no other agencies in the area are hiring, although some jobs may be available through a staffing pool or on a contingency basis. You must decide which of the following three employees to lay off. This is a nonunion agency, each of the nurses has the same number of years of service with the hospital, and all have had very similar job performance evaluations for the last three years.

Nurse A: Nancy is 50 years old and entered nursing later in life after raising a family of four. She is married to the hospital's chief of staff and some of the younger nurses on the unit resent her "country club" attitude. They think she is not really serious about nursing and only works to escape being bored. Nancy does a good job, but does have some difficulty working with other staff nurses. You personally like Nancy a great deal. She is closer to you in age and life experience than the other staff nurses, and you find yourself turning to her for advice and support. Nancy has confided in you that she really enjoys her newfound career. She says that for the first time in her life she has an identity of her own instead of always being somebody's daughter, spouse, or mother. Nancy has missed four days of work in the last six months, two times to take her mother to the doctor for evaluation of Alzheimer's disease, one because her husband unexpectedly told her that she had to accompany him to an important hospital social event, and one time she called in sick.

Nurse B: John is 35 years old and the only male nurse on your unit. He has suffered a great deal of personal crises and losses in the past two years. His 2-year-old son has Down syndrome, and his 10-year-old son was killed in an automobile accident last year. Six months ago his father died unexpectedly from a heart attack. John had confided in you that he is really struggling with these personal losses. He is especially having difficulty with losing his son because he says he will never be able to do all the "father/son" things with his 2-year-old son that would have been possible with the older son. John says he just doesn't feel the same kind of bond with either his 2-year-old son or his 6-year-old daughter. John also states that he's having difficulty with his wife. Their relationship is very strained and stressful. He's not sure if the marriage will survive. He says that he has been very depressed over all of these crises and has sought professional counseling. He also tells you in confidence that the psychiatrist has him on antidepressants to help him cope. John has missed four days of work in the last six months. All of them have been on Mondays. He says that the depression has at times made it difficult for him to start another week.

Nurse C: Carrie is 33 years old and very well liked by her peers. She is an informal leader in the group. You personally don't like Carrie very much. She was working on the unit before you became manager and she has constantly challenged you since you arrived. She is argumentative and resistant to change, but she always ends up doing what you have asked her to do. You worry about the effect that she has on unit morale. Yet you note that none of the staff nurses has ever reported having difficulties working with her. Nine months ago Carrie seriously injured her back when a patient she was ambulating started to fall. Carrie saved the patient from injury, but was on medical leave for six weeks because of the incident. Her recovery may have been hindered by the fact that she is 40 pounds overweight. Due to her back injuries, she often requests that she be assigned to Charge (desk) duty. Other staff nurses have offered to give her their Charge duty or volunteered to help her with patient care if she needs any assistance. Carrie has missed four days in the past six months, two days on two separate instances, both for complaints of back pain.

Which nurse will you lay off?

List two reasons to terminate or retain each of the nurses.

Nancy: 1.
       2.

John: 1.
       2.

Carrie: 1.
       2.

Indicate one personal, ethical, and legal issue that may be raised in terminating each of the three nurses.

Nancy: Personal:
       Ethical:
       Legal:

John: Personal:
       Ethical:
       Legal:

Carrie: Personal:
       Ethical:
       Legal:

ACTIVITY 19-4

ROLE STRESS

1. Write a short personal definition of the following terms:
   Role stress:

   Role ambiguity:

   Role conflict:

2. Write a brief report discussing stress in the workplace. Describe how it affects nurse managers personally, and how it affects the unit functioning. When preparing the report, consider the following concepts related to workplace stress:
   a) organizational factors leading to stress (e.g., job tasks, environment, supervisory styles)
   b) professional factors leading to stress (e.g., conflict over educational preparation, status of nursing in the health professions)
   c) interpersonal factors leading to stress (e.g., multiple roles, communication styles)
   d) individual factors leading to stress (e.g., personal problems, changes)
   e) societal factors leading to stress (e.g., economic factors, healthcare reform)
3. Analyze your current, personal level of stress, using a stress inventory such as the Social Readjustment Rating Scale. (Holmes and Rahe, 1967). (Note: You will not be required to share your personal stressors with faculty or other students as part of this assignment.)
4. Analyze your current work situation to determine the level of stress and/or reward that you receive from your employment. Use the chart below to identify factors that you regard as benefits or stressors in your current work situation.

PERCEIVED BENEFITS   **PERCEIVED STRESSORS**

ACTIVITY 19-5

MINDMAPPING

Devise a mindmap that depicts how personal and personnel problems may be exhibited in ways that are socially, legally, and professionally not sanctioned. Include personal and organizational factors that may intensify or inhibit substance abuse problems. Incorporate the roles of professional standards, agency policies, and procedures in controlling healthcare practitioners and safeguarding patients from unsafe practice.

REFERENCE

Holmes, T. & Rahe, R.H. (1967). The social readjustment rating scale. *Journal of Psychosomatic Research*, 1, 213-218.

PART 5

MANAGING CONSUMER CARE

CHAPTER 20

CONSUMER RELATIONSHIPS

Bonnie Nelson, M.S.N., R.N.

INTRODUCTION

It is essential to be aware of how consumer relations may affect the provision of nursing care. Consumers are faced with many changes in the healthcare field as well as in their interactions with the healthcare system when they are ill. It is difficult to allow someone else to control or influence what happens to you. When patients enter the hospital they lose a significant amount of control. The following exercises are to help you focus and identify how this loss of control might be reflected in what may seem to be very negative behaviors.

OBJECTIVES

- To describe how various members of the healthcare team can affect consumer relations.

- To apply the four major nursing responsibilities to a consumer relationship.

- To identify the feelings that may occur in both healthcare personnel and the consumer when a consumer has a complaint.

- To identify ways that consumer complaints may be handled.

- To use a transcultural assessment model to evaluate intercultural conflict.

Mr. Irons is transferred to your unit after having a myocardial infarction (MI). He is the C.E.O. at Interplast, an internationally known plastics manufacturer, specializing in healthcare supplies. In report it was noted that he has been very unhappy because of the limitations that have been placed on him in the ICU and is happy to go to the telemetry unit so that he can "carry on with his life." Mr. Irons has made arrangements for a laptop computer to be brought in and his secretary to be present for four hours a day. The staff has expressed concern regarding how wise it is for him to work while recovering from an MI and have witnessed many "type A" behaviors.

You are the nurse manager of the unit and when you return from a meeting you have a message to call the vice president for nursing regarding a patient complaint. When you call her, you are told that Mr. Irons has called the hospital administrator and demanded that a nurse on the unit be fired. You have been asked to investigate the situation.

Upon investigation you find that Mr. Irons is very upset because the nurse has been attempting to do some patient education regarding reducing stress and providing time for relaxation. He feels that he rests adequately at night and if he does not take care of business there will be serious consequences at his company. The staff nurse is upset and cries when approached, fearing being fired. The physician has ordered Valium for the patient.

Pages 396 through 405 in your textbook discuss four major nursing responsibilities to promote successful consumer relationships: service, advocacy, teaching, and leadership. Review these and answer the following questions.

1. How can your staff effectively provide services for Mr. Irons? List four ways.
   a)
   b)
   c)
   d)

2. If Mr. Irons refuses to collaborate with the staff in the provision of care and continues to be very directive, cite three effective ways to support staff regarding Mr. Irons' demands.
   a)
   b)
   c)

3. How are you going to respond to the vice president for nursing and to the hospital administration? Cite three critical areas to include in your response.
   a)
   b)
   c)

4. How will you handle Mr. Irons' demand for the staff nurse to be fired? Cite your approach and give supportive rationale for your selection.
   Approach

   Rationale

5. How will you be an advocate for Mr. Irons?
   Approach

   Rationale

In some institutions there are designated patient representatives who act as ombudsmen (advocates) for the hospital and the patient. (These persons may also be designated as "risk managers.") They are frequently first in line and highly skilled in handling patient complaints. Consider how a person in such a position may effectively respond to Mr. Irons concern? Make a list of at least three possible actions the patient representative could take.

1.

2.

3.

Compare your responses with at least two other classmates. Were your responses the same? Different? What would *you* do?

1.

2.

3.

Give rationale for each of these actions.

1.

2.

3.

ACTIVITY 20-3

(Refer to Activity 20-1.)

ROLE PLAY

Time limit: three to five minutes. Mr. Irons gives (not takes) orders and hasn't yet developed your listening skill.

1. Divide into small groups of five to seven students. Two students will role play while the others observe.

   Role players for Mr. Irons and the nurse: Don't be afraid to express feelings of anger, fear, or disappointment, etc. Think about how you would respond (both in words and in feelings) as if you were the person.

   Observers make notes about:

   a) what is said.

   b) what may be said differently.

   c) report on body language of the role players.

2. Discuss what was observed. (Note: Be open to make and receive recommendations regarding the nurse role play from your peers. This is your chance to receive nonthreatening feedback from your peers prior to confronting this possible situation clinically.)

3. *Role play repeat:* After completing one role play, two other members of the group rotate roles and complete the same process. Everyone should have the opportunity to have played at least one role, either nurse or patient.

   Possible role combinations: Mr. Irons and hospital administrator; nurse manager and vice president for nursing; Mr. Irons and nurse manager; nurse manager and staff nurse (the one Mr. Irons wants fired); nurse manager and Mr. Iron's physician; you, the ombudsman, and any one of the above.

4. Identify how it would feel to be in the role you are assigned. For example, as the staff nurse you may feel angry because you know what is best for Mr. Irons and how detrimental his behavior is to his health.

   I felt:

5. Discuss the feelings that were identified as a group. For example, as the nurse manager, while you were discussing the situation with the vice president for nursing you felt defensive.

   List five suggestions generated by the group to avoid defensiveness.

   a)

   b)

   c)

   d)

   e)

6. Consider what responses would have made you feel better. For example, you become angry while talking to Mr. Irons and tell him you are going to have his doctor talk to him. With the assistance of the group, list five ways that this might have been said differently.

   a)

   b)

   c)

   d)

   e)

ACTIVITY 20-4

It is the practice of some institutions to have patient care conferences. It is the goal of these conferences to handle problems that may occur and design a plan to provide quality care for the patient. It is also a good time to support your peers who may be having difficulties in providing care when there are problems.

You are responsible for leading a patient care conference and outlining a plan of care for Mr. Irons. Outline your plans for the conference. The patient should be involved in decisions made regarding the provision of care. Will you invite Mr. Irons to attend your patient care conference? Why? (Provide rationale.)

How will you involve Mr. Irons in his plan of care in the future? Identify five ways.

1.

2.

3.

4.

5.

ACTIVITY 20-5

(Refer to Activity 20-4)

Form a group of five to seven students and compare and discuss your individual responses. Develop group responses and provide rationale, using the space below to write out your rationale and plan in detail.

ACTIVITY 20-6

MINDMAPPING

Consider the interlocking roles of consumers and healthcare providers in achieving goals of optimum health. Develop a mindmap that incorporates the feelings and concerns of healthcare personnel and consumers when a complaint arises about the care provided. Include concepts related to transcultural concerns and role responsibilities of nurses and other healthcare workers in addressing concerns arising from complaints.

CHAPTER 21

CARE DELIVERY SYSTEMS

Bonnie Nelson, M.S.N., R.N.

INTRODUCTION

Various care delivery systems have evolved over time. Many were used successfully at first but later were abandoned as the financial concerns of the times demanded change. Also, one delivery system works better in one facility, while the same delivery system may not work in another facility. It is important to match the delivery system to the facility and to the financial constraints within which the system must function. It is also important to work within a system that promotes staff satisfaction.

OBJECTIVES

- To compare/contrast among five patient care delivery systems.

- To evaluate how potential management decisions may be unique in various care delivery systems.

- To design a care map for a specific patient population.

- To define how differentiated practice affects various members of the healthcare team as well as consumers.

ACTIVITY 21-1

You are the charge nurse on a ten-patient intermediate care unit. There are two RNs, one LPN, and one nursing assistant working today. Each care delivery system has different functions for care providers, e.g., in primary care, RNs have different functions than in functional systems. Describe the role of each care provider in each of the care delivery systems listed below.

Case Method

RN #1 role:

RN #2 role:

LPN role:

Nursing assistant role:

Functional

RN #1 role:

RN #2 role:

LPN role:

Nursing assistant role:

Team

RN #1 role:

RN #2 role:

LPN role:

Nursing assistant role:

Primary

RN #1 role:

RN #2 role:

LPN role:

Nursing assistant role:

Case Management

RN #1 role:

RN #2 role:

LPN role:

Nursing assistant role:

Additional considerations for the above exercise:

1. Cite two care delivery systems that would require a different staff mix (e.g., different number of RNs) to make it work?
   a)

   b)

2. As a B.S.N., which care delivery system would you be satisfied to work in? Cite reasons.

3. Which care delivery systems would your chief financial officer favor? Why?
   Favor:
   Rationale:

ACTIVITY 21-2

Form a group of three to five students and design and write a pamphlet describing the nursing care on the unit. Describe the functions of each member of the healthcare team for the consumer according to the type of care delivery system in your institution (refer to your descriptions in the preceding activity). Be certain that it is in terms that your clients (consumers) will understand and that it will attract them to the setting for which you are writing.

ACTIVITY 21-3

Refer to Exercise 21-2 in your textbook (p. 415) regarding the patient in pain (in a hospital using the functional method of care delivery).

1. Select three methods of care delivery that you prefer. Examine how a patient's concern might be addressed in each care delivery system.
   a) System:

   Patient concern:

   b) System:

   Patient concern:

   c) System:

   Patient concern:

2. Identify in each of the five delivery systems listed below where (in the institutional setting) delays in pain management can occur.
   Case Method:
   Functional:
   Team:
   Primary:
   Case Management:

3. As a manager, what would you do to deal with the issue of delay in treatment for at least three of the delivery systems. Be creative.
   a) System:

   Action:

   b) System:

   Action:

   c) System:

   Action:

ACTIVITY 21-4

Select a patient population that you have experience with and design a care map for that population. A care map is a way of identifying specific patient care outcomes on a daily basis. One advantage of determining a care map is to be able to make certain that patient activities and outcomes are timely, known to personnel, and beneficial to patients. A care map is also a good way to contain overall institutional costs by tracking length of stay.

Care Category	Day 1	Day 2	Day 3	Day 4
Consults				
Tests				
Treatments				
Medications				
Activity				
Nutrition				
D/C Plan				
Patient Variance				

ACTIVITY 21-5

Use the care map you designed in Activity 21-4 with a patient in your clinical setting. Use the following questions to guide your analysis: Did your patient follow the map or were there variances? If you had a variance, can you explain why? (Example: Patient developed an infection that delayed progress.)

Use the space below to write out your detailed analysis, giving specific examples of how your patient may have deviated from the map, any variances that occurred, and the like.

ACTIVITY 21-6

1. Using the comparison of roles of the technical and professional nurse found in the text in the box on page 429, discuss the role of different care providers according to their educational background.
   Graduate of:
   a) Associate degree program:

   b) Diploma program:

   c) Baccalaureate program:

2. Discuss how you think each care provider would react to this differentiation at the level of preparation held? As a B.S.N. student, does this feel fair to you? Why? Why not? List three reasons to support your position.
   a)

   b)

   c)

3. If you were the consumer, would you rather have a technical nurse or a professional nurse providing your care?

4. Do you think consumers know, understand, or care about the differences?
   Yes? No?
   Rationale:

5. Now that you have selected a position and provided rationale, cite two actions that you can take.
   a)

   b)

6. If you were the manager in an institution that has decided to adopt two levels of practice, how would you present this to the current staff?

MINDMAPPING

Devise a mindmap that incorporates the related concepts of different care delivery systems and differentiated practice of nurses. Incorporate how management decisions may vary with differing care delivery systems.

CHAPTER 22

PATIENT CLASSIFICATION, STAFFING, AND SCHEDULING

Bonnie Nelson, M.S.N., R.N.

INTRODUCTION

Staffing a nursing unit is a complex task. There are many things that must be considered when calculating the staffing needs of the unit you are managing. These include the average census of the unit, length of stay, patient classification, and staff mix. It is important to have a good understanding of the needs of the unit before attempting to determine the number and type of staff needed. Also consider the staff's needs and the personnel policies and contracts with the staff when planning the schedule.

OBJECTIVES:

- To calculate the number of staff required to operate a nursing unit.

- To complete a time schedule and identify potential problems.

- To identify issues and problems with self-scheduling.

- To write a set of rules for self-scheduling.

- To identify dilemmas inherent in managerial and staff self-scheduling.

- To identify and use a patient classification system.

You are the manager of a medical-surgical unit. The unit has thirty two beds and has an occupancy rate of 75 percent. It has been determined that there should be four RNs, two LPNs, and two nursing assistants on the day shift each day. There should be three RNs, one LPN and two nursing assistants on the afternoon shift, and three RNs, one LPN, and one nursing assistant on the night shift. Using the formulas from your textbook (pages 448-449), determine how many FTE's of each category employee will be necessary to cover the staffing requirements. (Remember, your unit is operating twenty four hours per day and all weekends and holidays.)

Your staff has the following allowed per contract:
    Seven holidays per year
    Ten sick days per year (funeral leaves deducted from sick time)
    Fifteen vacation days per year
All employees work every other weekend.

Determine:
    Number of RN FTE's needed
    Number of LPN FTE's needed
    Number of nursing assistant FTE's needed

Would you hire all full-time employees or would some part-time employees provide better coverage for your unit?
    Why?   Why not?
    Rationale:

Using this same staffing pattern determine what percentage of staff is allowed for each shift.
    _____ % allocated to 7 A.M. to 3 P.M.
    _____ % allocated to 3 P.M. to 11 P.M.
    _____ % allocated to 11 P.M. to 7 A.M.
    100 % Total

ACTIVITY 22-2

SCHEDULING

Using the same type of grid as represented on page 452 of your textbook (Figure 22-1), complete a unit staffing schedule for the 7 A.M. to 3 P.M. shift for a unit as described in Activity 22-1. (Suggest doing two weeks at least to establish weekend coverage.) Now consider the following revisions and constraints to your original planning.

1. What happens to the schedule if the second Monday is a holiday?

2. Include in the schedule one RN having a week of vacation time that includes her weekend to work.

3. Include a funeral leave (three consecutive days) for one LPN during the same time as the RN has vacation.

4. The staff is pushing for a change to twelve-hour shifts and working only three days per week. How does that affect your previous staffing and scheduling plans?
Staffing:

Scheduling:

5. In the space below, design a schedule for four weeks accommodating their request for twelve-hour days. Consider: would all of the staff be required to switch to twelve-hour shifts or would some be able to still work eight-hour shifts? (Remember, you do not need as much staff from 3 P.M. to 11 P.M.)

FOUR-WEEK SCHEDULE

SELF-SCHEDULING

You have called a staff meeting and have encouraged the staff to bring concerns regarding staff satisfaction. The meeting starts off with everyone wanting to start a self-scheduling program. Complete the following chart to illustrate and clarify the dilemmas, issues, and problems inherent in self-scheduling.

(+) Self-Scheduling	(+) Managerial Scheduling
1. Staff control over schedule	1. More efficient
2.	2.
3.	3.
4.	4.
5.	5.

(-) Self-Scheduling	(-) Managerial Scheduling
1. Negotiating with peers about schedule	1. Complaints from staff
2.	2.
3.	3.
4.	4.
5.	5.

Before starting self-scheduling you would need to write some guidelines. Identify four more that you believe are necessary to incorporate as you develop the new schedule. Review the chart above.

1. May only schedule Friday off with your weekend one time per month.

2.

3.

4.

5.

ACTIVITY 22-4

PATIENT CLASSIFICATION

1. Identify the patient classification instrument used at your institution. Request a copy of one from your clinical faculty member to use to complete this exercise. Bring a copy to class and share with a classmate from a different institution.

2. Cite two similarities and differences between each form.
   Similarities:
   a)

   b)

   Differences:
   a)

   b)

3. Compare the use of a patient classification instrument with at least two patients. Identify how the use of it differs for each patient.
   a)

   b)

MINDMAPPING

Create a mindmap depicting the interrelationships among staffing, scheduling, and patient classifications systems. Incorporate potential competing concerns involved in mangerial and in staff self-scheduling.

PART 6

MANAGING PERSONAL RESOURCES

CHAPTER 23

ROLE TRANSITION

Joseph B. Hurst, Ph.D., Ed.D., and Ann W. Baker, Ph.D., R.N.

INTRODUCTION

Chapter 23 of the textbook presents a long list of roles, responsibilities, and aspects of a nurse management position. Making the transition is discussed in depth and compared to the building of an intimate relationship. New managers often flounder around in their new roles because although they usually are great caregivers and doers, their new position demands much more than that. Stepping into these new roles and responsibilities, with all the associated accountability, involves a great deal of change, adapting, and learning. Throughout your textbook, much has been said about changing your behavior, leading others, managing change, and creating new procedures. This chapter promotes your own assessment of the many roles a manager plays, others' expectations and the conflicts inherent in them, and your own "readiness" for managing. It also includes a tool to help you assess how you tend to take risks and the factors that support and block your taking risks.

OBJECTIVES

- To clarify and assess the many roles associated with nurse management positions.

- To determine one's own readiness for or level of satisfaction in a nurse management position.

- To assess the degree to which you take risks and the personal and environmental factors that affect your risk taking.

- To analyze short case examples and determine how you might take appropriate risks and/or support others in doing so.

- To analyze the degree to which groups might be more or less supportive of risks and how a manager could promote appropriate levels of risk taking by others.

ACTIVITY 23-1

1. Read Chapter 23 in the textbook and complete the "Roles Assessment" on pages 466-467. In that assessment you are asked to analyze job responsibilities, opportunities to contribute and grow professionally, lines of communication, and expectations of others around the nurse manager. Talk to two staff nurses and ask each of them, "What are the two most important roles that a nurse manager must fulfill?"

a1)

a2)

b1)

b2)

Ask a nurse manager, "What are the two most important roles that you must fulfill?"

a)

b)

Compare the responses:

Similarities:

Differences:

Conflicts:

Share your responses with two or three others in your class. Now what do all of you conclude about:

Similarities:

Differences:

Conflicts:

Discuss responses with your classmates and others (managers, staff) and have them assist in clarifying the multiple roles and expectations.

2. Create a mindmap of the roles assessment results including your thoughts and observations. What roles and responsibilities excite you? Why?

Which ones seem to demand a "risk and stretch" for you? Why?

Which roles and responsibilities would you rather not have? Why?

ACTIVITY 23-2

Complete the self-assessment in your textbook on page 474. As it asks, talk with a mentor of yours and compare your perspective on yourself with the mentor's perspective. You also could use some of the sentence completions below as additional items on which to focus.

1. One recent example of my success in providing leadership is

2. I'm especially proud of my ability to

3. The part of my job I especially like is

4. I believe in my capability to manage difficult

5. I'm very responsible in relation to

6. A goal I've met in the past year of which I'm most proud is

7. I think my supervisor would evaluate my effectiveness as

8. My colleagues would describe me as

9. I accomplish the most when I

10. One thing I'm more successful with this year is

1. Think about relationships that you have had difficulty developing and maintaining. What could you learn about role transition from what you did and did not do in those relationships?

   What could you apply to future role transitions?

2. List at least two typical conflicts between your personal expectations and an immediate supervisor's expectations.

   a)

   b)

   How can you resolve this conflict in a way that your relationship with the supervisor improves?

ACTIVITY 23-4

Role transition most often involves some degree of risk taking. This exercise can help you discover your own risk-taking style and expand your ability to use it intentionally. Use the space provided to write your answers to the questions below.

1. What is risk taking? What affects the degree to which you tend to take risks?

2. How can you support others in taking appropriate risks? How can you get that same kind of support for yourself and others?

3. How and when does your risk taking have to change depending on the situations in which you find yourself as a manager? Why?

4. What new behaviors could you incorporate into your risk-taking style?

ACTIVITY 23-5

MINDMAPPING

After reading Chapter 23 in the textbook and completing the activities in this workbook, develop a mindmap that depicts your perceptions about the roles, responsibilities, expectations, interpersonal interactions, environmental factors, and risk-taking behaviors, and conflicts inherent in managerial positions. Be certain to include your interpretations of essential behaviors and responsibilities of the managerial role so that this may be a guide to view the position from your perspective and that of others.

CHAPTER 24

POWER, POLITICS, AND INFLUENCE

Ann W. Baker, Ph.D., R.N.

INTRODUCTION

Who would you say is the most important person at your hospital? Give it some thought before you respond! Is it the president or chief executive officer? Is it the person who makes the most money? Is it the person who supervises the most employees? Is it the person who has the authority to fire or demote you? Or the physician with the most influence? Is it the patient who threatens to sue you? This chapter examines the nature, impact, and uses of power in nursing management.

OBJECTIVES

- To identify the different sources of personal and professional power.

- To analyze situations involving power and determine the use, misuse, and "missed opportunities" observed.

- To compare and contrast the essential attributes of nursing and non-nursing professionals.

- To identify misuses, missed opportunities, and appropriate uses of power.

ACTIVITY 24-1

1. Review the definitions of power in the box on page 482 of your textbook (Types of Social Power). Write a short personal example fitting each definition:

   1. Expert:

   2. Information:

   3. Legitimate:

   4. Coercive:

   5. Reward:

   6. Referent:

   7. Connection:

2. Now reread the introduction to this chapter. Who is the most powerful person at your hospital? Why could it be you, the nurse?

Read the case below, considering the different types of power. Reflect on the behaviors listed for Debbie, the emergency department charge nurse in the case.

CLINICAL CASE STUDY

Debbie Starr (R.N., C.E.N.) the charge nurse in a very busy emergency department, was exhausted at the end of her twelve-hour shift. Sixty-six patients had been triaged, assessed, cared for, counseled, educated, admitted, transferred, and/or discharged. One patient died. Some of the nursing responsibilities/behaviors carried out by Debbie on this shift included:

a) took/gave shift report every four hours.

b) assigned staff to patient care responsibilities.

c) assigned staff to nonnursing responsibilities such as ordering supplies, room checks, and testing emergency equipment.

d) oriented two new medical students to department protocols and expectations.

e) requested assistance from the nursing supervisor to obtain ICU beds for two critical patients.

f) called the children's protective agency to request emergency placement for three abandoned children brought in by the police.

g) yelled over the phone at a newspaper reporter who insisted upon obtaining details of a recent accident.

h) assisted a staff nurse to support very distressed family members whose elderly parent had just died.

i) talked to the coroner for ten minutes by phone.

j) cared for five patents whose nurse left for his dinner break.

k) assisted three staff members who were restraining an out-of-control inebriated patient.

l) intervened between a staff nurse and physician who disagreed about a patient care issue.

m) promised to talk privately to an angry unit secretary later in the shift if there was time.

n) gathered all staff together at 11 P.M. to thank them for their hard work and good care.

Write out short responses to the following questions about the case.

1. Cite all of the bases of power that Debbie exhibited. (Place the number of the power base that she used at the left side of each statement above.) Label each one according to the chapter definition: 1, expert; 2, information; 3, legitimate; 4, coercive; 5, reward; 6, referent; and 7, connection.

2. How did this nurse empower the staff? Cite two ways.
   a)
   b)

3. Cite two missed opportunities for empowerment that you saw.
   a)

   b)

4. Visualize this nurse and write a description of her.
   What does she look like?

   How does she speak to people?

   What values does she embody?

What influential person in your life does she remind you of?

ACTIVITY 24-3

Empowerment as defined in Chapter 24 in the textbook is the "process by which we facilitate the participation of others in decision making and taking action in an environment where there is an equitable distribution of power." Empowerment is power sharing and a form of feminine/feminist leadership. All of the following can be powerful attributes of a professional nurse. Rank them in order of importance to you by numbering them in the blanks provided (1 being most important).

___ a) professional knowledge, specialized knowledge
___ b) technological competence
___ c) professional experience
___ d) problem-solving skills
___ e) comfort with conflict resolution
___ f) ability to communicate clearly with colleagues
___ g) a commitment to organizational philosophy and mission
___ h) above-average financial compensation
___ i) a sense of humor
___ j) positive feelings of job satisfaction

Give this same list to a nursing colleague and to a nonnursing colleague and ask them to rank these items. Compare all three rankings. What similarities and differences exist?

Similarities:

Differences:

ACTIVITY 24-4

1. Meet in groups of three or four. Discuss the responses you wrote for the questions about the case in Activity 24-2 featuring Debbie Starr, RN.

2. What "power tools" were most effective in this example?

   a)

   b)

   c)

   d)

3. Describe the "coalition building" behaviors Debbie demonstrated.

   a)

   b)

   c)

4. Discuss the following assertion and its implication for your future in nursing and in nursing management: "Collegiality demands mutual respect, not friendship!" (Chapter 24, page 490). Are friendship and being a respected manager mutually exclusive? Why or why not?

ACTIVITY 24-5

Meet in groups of five or six. Combine your group rankings from Activity 24-3. (Or make arrangements to combine the entire class's rankings.)

1. What conclusions can you draw from this exercise? Identify, describe, and explain differences that exist among the rankings by nurses?
   a)

   b)

   c)

2. What can you conclude?
   a)

   b)

   c)

3. Do differences exist between the nurse rankings and the nonnurse rankings? Discuss specific similarities, differences, and conclusions.
   Similarities:
   a)

   b)

   Differences:
   a)

   b)

   Conclusions:
   a)

   b)

ACTIVITY 24-6

MINDMAPPING

Devise a mindmap that depicts the associations among the sources, uses, misuses, and "missed opportunities" inherent in the potential of personal and professional power.

CHAPTER 25

STRESS MANAGEMENT: A BALANCING ACT

Joseph B. Hurst, Ph.D., Ed.D.

INTRODUCTION

If you are like many people in your profession, you feel a great deal of stress and are usually more concerned about others' health and well-being than your own! Can you change your beliefs and habits enough to reduce stress and unproductivity while increasing challenge, growth, and tranquillity in your life? This chapter focuses on ways to balance the stimulation (neutral meaning of stress) and tranquillity polarity in the important areas of your life. Professional people need to manage this polarity competently and intentionally within their work and nonwork lives. We need to have "equal" elements of challenge, excitement, and accomplishment, on the one hand, and peace, relaxation, and renewal, on the other, in both our personal and professional lives.

OBJECTIVES

- **To determine the major factors triggering distress, eustress, boredom, and renewal, and the typical physical, emotional, and cognitive reactions to each.**

- **To compare and contrast your actual degree of balance of stimulation and tranquillity in the personal, school, and work/clinical domains of your life with an "ideal" balance.**

- **To develop and revise a plan of action regarding stress.**

ACTIVITY 25–1

1. Read Chapter 25 in the textbook. Write out the stress plan suggested in Exercises 27-6 and 27-7 on page 510.
2. Study the stimulation/tranquillity diagram in Figure 25-1 below.
   a) Notice that there are positive, healthy outcomes of being stimulated in life (the "eustress" quadrant). In what activities are you engaged (or could you be) that lead to these results in your clinical/work life? In your school life? In your personal life? Write these activities and the results of engaging in them in the appropriate sections of the charts on page 257 of this workbook.
   b) Notice in the polarity diagram in Figure 25-1 that when you overdo these kind of activities (and have negative judgments about your ability to cope effectively with them all) there are negative consequences in the "stress" quadrant. Now in the charts, list the activities (including judgments) that trigger these negative results and the actual results you experience in your clinical/work life? In your school life? In your personal life?

L+	STRESS AND TRANQUILLITY POLARITY	R+
EUSTRESS • Exhilaration, Thrill, Enthusiasm • Challenge; Bold View of Life • New Goals and Priorities • Growth and Transformation • Accomplishment and Contribution • Creativity and Experimentation • Issues are Confronted		**RENEWAL** • Relaxation, Peace • Lack of Stress Disorders • Calmness, Patience • Replenishment, Rejuvenation • Sensed being "centered" • Freedom and Spontaneity
STRESS • Overwhelm, Worry, Anxiety • Stress-Related Disorders • Irritation, Impatience • Exhaustion, Burnout • Sense of Burden, Overcommitment • Feelings of Entrapment **DISTRESS**		**TRANQUILLITY** • Stuckness, Apathy, Disinterest • Boredom; Static View of Life • Status Quo • No Growth and Transformation • Accomplishment and Contribution • Rigid Passivity, Depression • Avoidance of Issues **BOREDOM**
L-		R-

Figure 25-1
Hurst, Joe "Stress and Tranquillity Polarity, "Paper presented at polarity forum, University of Toledo, 11/12/93.

c) The "renewal" quadrant tranquillity side of this diagram has very positive, healthy benefits. Look at the positive consequences in the diagram and list renewing activities and results in all three areas of your life in the charts.

d) The "tranquillity" quadrant of the polarity diagram represents *boredom* and feeling unproductive. People often short–change opportunities for tranquillity and renewal because of a perception of boredom or of becoming involved in activities that are a "waste of time." Add your current activities and results to the charts.

BALANCING THE STIMULATION/TRANQUILLITY CONTROVERSY

CLINICAL/WORK		SCHOOL/EDUCATIONAL	
Present Activities	Results	Present Activities	Results
+		+	
-		-	
New Activities	Results	New Activities	Results
+		+	
-		-	

PERSONAL LIFE

Present Activities	Results
+	+
-	-
New Activities	Results
+	+
-	-

3. Now your charts for each area of your life are complete. Look at the degree to which you are balanced and out of balance. The diagrams in Figure 25-2 and 25-3 on pages 259 and 260 illustrate balanced and unbalanced management of this dilemma. One key to imbalance is the degree to which you experience negative results in any area and where you try to have either challenge or tranquillity in one area and the other in another area. For example, if you challenge yourself at work and school, and then try to get all your tranquillity at home, you are out of balance. Draw a set of lines that represent your flow from one hemisphere to the other in each area (see Chapter 17 in the text and the chart on page 259 of this workbook).

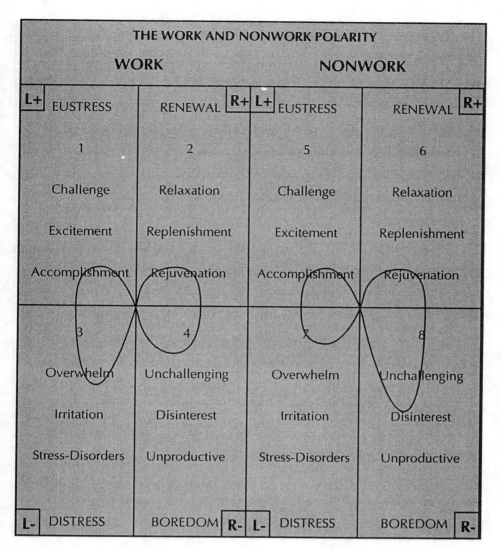

THE WORK AND NONWORK POLARITY

WORK		NONWORK	
L+ EUSTRESS	RENEWAL **R+**	**L+** EUSTRESS	RENEWAL **R+**
1	2	5	6
Challenge	Relaxation	Challenge	Relaxation
Excitement	Replenishment	Excitement	Replenishment
Accomplishment	Rejuvenation	Accomplishment	Rejuvenation
3	4	7	8
Overwhelm	Unchallenging	Overwhelm	Unchallenging
Irritation	Disinterest	Irritation	Disinterest
Stress-Disorders	Unproductive	Stress-Disorders	Unproductive
L- DISTRESS	BOREDOM **R-**	**L-** DISTRESS	BOREDOM **R-**

Figure 25-2 Unbalanced Results.

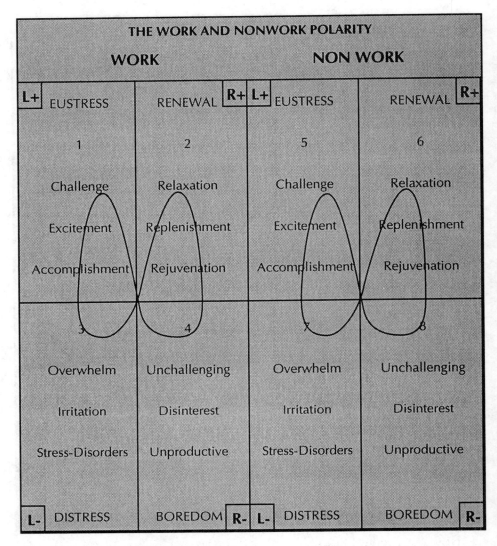

Figure 25-3 Balanced Polarity Results.
Adapted from B. Johnson (1992). *Polarity Management.*

ACTIVITY 25–2

Review Chapter 25 in your textbook, the stress plan from Activity 25–1/item 1 above, the charts from that same activity, and any other resources you have about stress. Add to your stress plan so that it is balanced in your personal, professional, and educational life. You will need to address these questions:

1. What present practices support and block my shifting from side to side in my work, school and personal life? What new practices would promote flexible shifting between sides. Write your answers in the "Force-Field Analysis of Stress Controversy" below.
Support

Block

2. How can I add tranquillity to my clinical/work and school activities?

By when

3. How can I add excitement, challenge, and peace to my personal life?

By when

4. How can I reduce distress, feelings of being overwhelmed, and unproductiveness from all three areas?

By when?

5. How could I assist others around me in being more balanced and by when?

FORCE–FIELD ANALYSIS OF STRESS CONTROVERSY
WORK/CLINICAL

Blocking Forces Preventing
Shifting from Pole to Pole

Supporting Forces Promoting
Shifting from Pole to Pole

New Possibilities To Increase Appropriate Shifting Between Poles

SCHOOL/EDUCATIONAL

Blocking Forces Preventing
Shifting Between Poles

Supporting Forces Promoting
Shifting Between Poles

New Possibilities To Increase Appropriate Shifting Between Poles

PERSONAL LIFE

Blocking Forces Preventing
Shifting Between Poles

Supporting Forces Promoting
Shifting Between Poles

New Possibilities To Increase Appropriate Shifting Between Poles

ACTIVITY 25–3

1. List suggestions for reducing negative symptoms of a) stimulation (distress) and tranquillity (boredom) while increasing the b) beneficial results of stimulation (eustress) and tranquillity (peace and renewal).

   a)

   b)

2. In a small group or with the entire class, discuss real-life examples of imbalances and balances in these areas and items from your stress plans above in Activity 25-1. Pinpoint major blocks, supports, and new actions.

   Supports:

   Blocks:

   New actions:

MINDMAPPING

Generate a mindmap for yourself that depicts interrelationships among personal and professional sources of stress, strategies for stress reduction, and techniques for successful balancing of stress and eustress.

CHAPTER 26

CAREER MANAGEMENT

Mary J. Keenan, Ph.D., R.N., Mary Beth Hayward, M.S.N., R.N., and Joseph B. Hurst, Ph.D., Ed.D.

INTRODUCTION

Career planning/mapping is a broader activity than finding a job. Many people move from job to job without reflection, goals, and plans for the future. This chapter identifies ways to strengthen both the personal and professional aspects of your life as a nurse through career planning and mapping and by focusing on your career aspirations and possibilities. The emphasis is on being the artist who paints your future life on canvas, or the author who writes your autobiography.

OBJECTIVES

* To help you identify your career goals and aspirations, both short- and long-term.

* To explore strategies for a self-directed approach to career planning and control.

* To apply career management theory to the development of a career path.

ACTIVITY 26–1

SELF–ASSESSMENT

Before completing the activities in this chapter, take a few moments to reflect on the questions that follow. Write your answers in the spaces provided.

1. Do you think of yourself as prospective nurse manager, clinical specialist, advanced practice nurse, nurse practitioner?

2. Do you see yourself as being in charge of your future?

3. How would you describe your career development at this time?

4. How would you describe your career development now?

5. What are your short–term goals?

6. What are your long-term goals?

7. What would you like to be doing after graduation?

   Five years from now?

   Ten years from now?

   Twenty five years from now?

8 Are you seriously considering the nursing profession with a clear view of the type of position you would like to obtain in the near and distant future?

9 What additional education, skills, and credentials do you need? What is your network?

ACTIVITY 26–2

BUILDING A CAREER PLAN

1. Stating your career aspiration in writing is a vital step, even though at this time it may be only a dream. Nevertheless, it can serve as a guiding force in your life, and all of the succeeding goals that you write may contribute to it. What is your overall goal?

2. List three specific measurable goals that you can aspire to in the next three years.
   a)
   b)
   c)
   List three goals for the next five years.
   a)
   b)
   c)
   You should continue this process throughout your professional career and life.

3. List three contributions that you feel most satisfied about making to the lives of others.
   a)
   b)
   c)

4. List the group(s) of people to whom you are committed and to whom you make the contributions you listed in item 3 above (e.g., promoting mobility and independence in the elderly). Don't forget your family and friends.
   a)
   b)
   c)

5. List the "benefits" you want from your position/career. Consider both personal and professional benefits. Add to the list below:
   financial security   autonomy   clinical specialty
   affiliation   achievement

6. Make an appointment to "shadow" someone in a position to which you aspire. Develop a list of objectives for the time you spend observing this person. Share this list with the person, and plan to schedule a short conference with him/her to share and gain feedback about your observations, goals, aspirations, and insights.
   Objectives:
   a)
   b)
   c)
   d)
   e)
   Choosing a position and developing a career also involves matching your talents, beliefs, and goals with your aspirations. List some specific questions to ask about the work the person does, and what special things you should observe. Share something about yourself, and request feedback if you sense

that you and the person/position are a good match.

Questions to ask:

a)

b)

c)

d)

e)

Special things to observe:

a)

b)

c)

d)

e)

7. With another student from your class, make a list of several typical questions that might be asked at an interview.

a)

b)

c)

d)

e)

f)

g)

h)

With the same classmate, select four of these questions and practice answering them. Write your answers in the spaces provided.

a)

b)

c)

d)

Activity 26-6 in this chapter explains how to do a job interview role play to give you further preparation for your actual job interviews.

8. Make a list of personal contacts whom you could use for reference or possible referrals for positions. Whom might they know? Who are others in your "network" that could provide information about, and professional referrals for, job possibilities? List at least five sources of job information (e.g., career/job fairs, newspaper ads, etc.) and career opportunities. Spend time looking at, reading, and/or collecting several of these sources. What trends have you discovered?

Personal Contacts for Reference/Referrals	Other Contacts Whom They Might Know

Other Possible Sources of Information/Professional Referrals

Five Sources of Job Information
a)

b)

c)

d)

e)

Trends You Have Discovered

ACTIVITY 26–3

As graduation time approaches, you need to think about where to apply for your next job. You also need to think about the future. Review your responses in the previous activity and build upon them in this exercise.

"Where do I start?" With all the changes in healthcare and nursing and the developments in healthcare reform, you need to start on a course that will carry you forward into 2025. The questions and activities outlined below can assist you in formulating your directions now.

1. Select an area that interests you, one that you like and would enjoy learning more about.

2. Find nursing publications in the area that you have selected above, for example, magazines or journals such as *American Journal of Nursing, Nursing and Health Care, Critical Care Nursing*. Read the editorials from the last four months and the table of contents to determine the main areas of focus in the domain that you have selected:
   a)
   b)
   c)
   d)
   e)
3. Interview one or two professional nurses practicing in the area that you have selected. Ask the questions below (plus additional ones of your choosing) and record the interviewees' answers in the space provided:
   a) How did you happen to select this area?

   b) What skills do you believe are critical for nurses practicing in this area?

   c) What changes have you seen occur in this area and in your practice since you have been in it?

   d) What do you believe will be changes that will occur in two years? Five years?

4. Seek information about career opportunities from a professional organization in the area that you have selected (e.g., American Nurses Association, American Association of Critical Care Nurses, American Organization of Nurse Executives). Describe your findings in the space below.

5. What do all of these sources say in common about how to prepare and pursue a career in the area? Where do they differ? What seems to be the basis for the differences?

6. Seek out at least two other students in class who have interests similar to yours. Share and discuss your information. In the space below, generate a plan for yourself that includes both advanced education and clinical development.

7. What are the certification requirements in the area that you have selected?

ACTIVITY 26–4

PREDICAMENT: SELECTING THE "RIGHT" POSITION

You have submitted applications and résumés to several area hospitals. On Monday the nurse recruiter at Happy Days Hospital telephones and offers you a float position on nights at the hospital. You are overjoyed but request a few days to consider accepting the position immediately. On Tuesday the head nurse on 6 East at the same hospital telephones and offers you a position on nights. The latter position is very appealing as you know the staff on the unit and feel they would be supportive of you. However, a float position will provide opportunities for nursing practice in different specialties. Nevertheless, you would really like to continue your education and pursue your M.S.N. in a defined specialty area that you have decided on. The university is fifteen miles away, very prestigious, and offers the specialty that you desire. It accepts part-time students, and you have applied and been admitted. What do you do, now that you have at least three options from which to select? Outline your plan for decision making.

1. List the pros and cons of each position.

FLOAT POSITION

Pros	Cons
a)	a)
b)	b)
c)	c)
d)	d)
e)	e)

6 EAST POSITION

Pros	Cons
a)	a)
b)	b)
c)	c)
d)	d)
e)	e)

2. How do the positions fit with your career goals that you have mapped in Activity 26-1?

3. Which position will give the direction and supervision you need at this point in your career?

4. Can you work the hours required in each of the positions? What is your own personal "prime time" of day/night to take advantage of your optimal energy level?

5. How do the demands of the positions fit with your graduate school schedule?

6. What are the networking possibilities in each of the positions?

7. How will this choice influence your career in five, ten, etc. years?

ACTIVITY 26–5

You are a nurse manager at Happy Days Hospital. Census has been very low for months and rumors abound about downsizing the institution. You have a B.S.N. with seven years of nursing experience (three years in management). Outline a career plan to increase your marketability for other positions.

1. What course of action could you take at this time to be prepared for change?

2. What additional knowledge /skills will you need to acquire to assume a new position?

3. What is the strategic plan for Happy Days Hospital?

4. How can you prepare yourself to contribute to this plan and assume a new position?

5. Should you look elsewhere for a position that will use your knowledge and expertise?

6. What suggestions do those in your network have about altering your career pathway?

7. List three alternatives open to you, showing both the pros and cons.
   Alternative
   Pros:

   Cons:

   Alternative
   Pros:

   Cons:

   Alternative
   Pros:

   Cons:

JOB INTERVIEW ROLE PLAY

This activity gives you an opportunity to pair up with a classmate and take turns role playing a job interview situation. Each of you will have an opportunity to be both interviewer and interviewee, and to give each other feedback.

Pre–Role Play Preparation

1. Review the Appendix to Chapter 26 in your textbook, particularly the material on page 538 entitled "Questions to Ask/to be Asked," and select questions to use in the interview.
2. Develop a position description for the job that is to be filled, or choose one from an actual advertised position. (This is the position for which you will be interviewed.)
3. Bring your résumé, list of interview questions, and position description to class to use during the role play.

Role Play

1. Choose a partner with whom to perform the role play.
2. Exchange your interview questions, position descriptions, and résumés. Spend a few minutes studying these materials to familiarize yourself with them. Add at least two other challenging questions to your classmate's list of interview questions, to see how she/he responds to the unexpected.
3. Draw straws or flip a coin to decide who goes first to be interviewed.
4. Sitting face to face with your partner, conduct a short (ten to fifteen minute) interview.
5. After each interview is over, give each other feedback about how each of you interviewed and how you might improve in the future.

ACTIVITY 26–7

MINDMAPPING

Create a scenario that represents a mindmap of strategies and opportunities that can assist you in taking charge of your career and your future.